Doctor–patient Communication in Chinese and Western Medicine

Drawing on naturally occurring doctor–patient conversations in real-life medical consultations, this book analyzes the similarities and differences in doctor–patient communication and patient satisfaction between traditional Chinese medicine (TCM) and Western medicine (WM) practiced in China.

Little research is available looking at WM being practiced in Asian countries, and misunderstanding about Eastern medicines such as TCM can result in unwarranted claims and suspicions. This volume contributes to research on doctor–patient communication by exploring the communication behaviors between doctors and older patients who are able to communicate independently in both TCM and WM practiced in mainland China and evaluating patient satisfaction with their medical experiences. The book reports findings and insights from three independent and methodologically diverse studies, drawing on data from 69 real-life medical consultations: 30 from TCM and 39 from WM. Using conversation analysis, the Roter Interaction Analysis System, and both quantitative and qualitative methods, Ying Jin examines the differences between TCM and WM to help reveal the dynamics of doctor–patient interactions, the contextual details, and the impact of the clinical culture on medical communication. This insightful book will appeal to scholars and students from linguistics, language, and health communication as well as medical practitioners interested in doctor–patient communication and intercultural communication.

The findings reported here will shine a light on the relationship between clinical differences, health communication, and patient outcomes.

Ying Jin received her PhD degree from the Department of English, the Hong Kong Polytechnic University. She is currently involved in several international collaborations in areas such as stigma communication and patient-centeredness. Her major research interests include sociolinguistics, health communication, and workplace discourse.

Routledge Studies in Language, Health and Culture

Series Editor: Olga Zayts,
University of Hong Kong, Hong Kong

This series has several distinctive features. First, it investigates health communication through linguistic lenses. The contributions to the series in the form of research monographs or targeted edited volumes will introduce the readers to a range of linguistic approaches, including, but not limited to (critical) discourse analysis, sociolinguistics, multimodal analysis, corpus analysis, conversation analysis, and so on. Second, what will bring these versatile approaches together in the series is that they will draw on authentic empirical data from a range of healthcare contexts (e.g., acute care, traditional medicine, secondary care), going beyond the traditional doctor–patient encounters and expanding the focus of inquiry to online healthcare provision, interprofessional communication, and so on.

Second, the series focuses specifically on contexts outside of the mainstream English-dominant healthcare contexts. The series solicits proposals from contributors working on healthcare communication in the Asia-Pacific, South America, continental Europe, and so on, putting to the forefront the growing body of research representing versatile sociocultural and linguistic contexts.

Third, it is expected that some contributions will focus on multicultural and multilingual healthcare encounters, thus making the series of relevance to a broad readership around the world.

In line with some of the core principles of linguistic research in healthcare contexts, the series will encourage contributions that, in addition to advancing the linguistic field, will also stress relevance to professional practice (Sarangi and Candlin, 2011). The editor will invite, where appropriate, healthcare and medical professionals in a relevant field to critically review and endorse, or to write a short foreword to the contributions. This feature will encourage a transdisciplinary dialogue between linguistic and health communication scholars and healthcare and medical professionals, thus increasing the potential readership.

Doctor–Patient Communication in Chinese and Western Medicine
Ying Jin

For more details on the series, please visit: www.routledge.com/Routledge-Studies-in-Language-Health-and-Culture/book-series/RSLHC

Doctor–patient Communication in Chinese and Western Medicine

Ying Jin

Routledge
Taylor & Francis Group

LONDON AND NEW YORK

First published 2022
by Routledge
4 Park Square, Milton Park, Abingdon, Oxon OX14 4RN

and by Routledge
605 Third Avenue, New York, NY 10158

Routledge is an imprint of the Taylor & Francis Group, an Informa business

© 2022 Ying Jin

British Library Cataloguing-in-Publication Data
A catalogue record for this book is available from the British Library

Library of Congress Cataloguing-in-Publication Data
A catalog record has been requested for this book

ISBN: 978-0-367-75307-8 (hbk)
ISBN: 978-0-367-75309-2 (pbk)
ISBN: 978-1-00-316192-9 (ebk)

DOI: 10.4324/9781003161929

Typeset in Galliard
by Newgen Publishing UK

Dedication

To my parents

for always loving and supporting me

Contents

Figures

Tables

Acknowledgments

I wish to express my utmost gratitude to my supervisors, Dr. Dennis Tay, Prof. Bernadette Watson, and Prof. Stephen Evans (who has peacefully passed away) for your professional support and guidance and constant care throughout the research process. Your critical comments have contributed insights on my readings of the data from divergent perspectives.

I wish to express my deepest gratitude to Dr. Dennis Tay, my chief supervisor, for your guidance and direction throughout the entire course of this research project. Thank you for your wisdom and vision at each of the critical junctures of my study. Your unwavering support has brought me courage and confidence in the completion of this book.

I am also indebted to Prof. Bernadette Watson, my co-supervisor, for bridging my knowledge gap on medical communication. Your expertise as a psychologist has brought me insights and alternative viewpoints on the reading of the data and understanding of the meaning potential behind discourse.

Special thanks also go to Prof. Stephen Evans, my prior co-supervisor, for your support and help during my first year of study. Your motivation as a scholar always encouraged me to work harder. May you rest in peace!

1 Medical coexistence

1.1 Overview: communication and medicine

> *Yin-yang* is the law of the universe, the governing principle of myriad things and the parent [origin] of all changes, the ultimate cause of life and death, the hall of residence of the mind (*shenming*). Prior to treating a disease, seek [try to understand] its origin first.
>
> (Kong, 2010, p. 217)

Over the years, scholars have consistently agreed upon the centrality of communication in interpersonal relationships. This is particularly the case in service encounters where providers need to know their clients' dos and don'ts to serve them. Things are more complicated in medical encounters where the client (the patient) usually comes with a dual pursuit for both care and cure. Through communication, providers and patients exchange their interpretations of the meaning of illness (i.e., what is wrong with the patient) and the meaning of disease (i.e., what is wrong with the body) (Reading, 1977). While the therapeutic power of medicine is indisputable, studies have also reported the immense therapeutic power of communication (Street, 2013; Williams et al., 1998). It is widely endorsed that the art of communication and the art of medicine are intricately crafted together to achieve both therapeutic and interpersonal goals. The implications of this claim for the relationship between communication and health have triggered a great deal of research, applying knowledge from linguistics, psychology, and sociology to understand the intricate dynamics between health and language. Linguists are interested in furthering our understanding of the use of language or language-related activities (e.g., questions, utterance-final particles, small talk). Psychologists focus their efforts primarily on the underlying motives that could explain the communication behaviors between health professionals and clients (e.g., to accommodate or highlight intergroup differences). Sociologists are particularly attentive to the social structures reflected in medical discourse. The divergent yet complementary research focuses have yielded exciting interdisciplinary research in health communication. The present study is one such research borrowing knowledge from both linguistics and sociology to expand

DOI: 10.4324/9781003161929-1

the understanding of doctor–patient communication in two clinically different encounters in China.

1.2 Medical coexistence in China

1.2.1 Chinese medicine: traditions, theories, and therapeutic methods

Before the introduction of Western medicine (WM) into China in the early 1800s (Anderson, 2006), Chinese medicine (or traditional Chinese medicine, TCM) was the only therapeutic method to treat patients in old China. It is documented that the earliest extant contribution of TCM, *Huangdi neijing* (Inner Classic of the Yellow Emperor), was written thousands of years ago, between 300 BCE and 100 BCE, and is still regarded as a great authority. The Classic describes the diagnosis, treatments, and preventions of a range of diseases and provides suggestions for a healthy lifestyle, which conforms well with the current practice of chronic disease prevention (Hesketh & Zhu, 1997). While a detailed explanation of how TCM works is beyond the scope of this book, a brief overview of the etiology and pathology that guide TCM will help us better understand the differences in TCM and WM, making a case for our study.

To many WM professionals, TCM treats patients using a system of interpretation that is difficult to understand (for more discussion, see Cai, 1988). Key to TCM is the cosmic theory of yin-yang, which posits that the universe is a complete whole consisting of two complementary opposites (Lao et al., 2012). The concepts of *yin* (negative) and *yang* (positive) are used to describe the universe, for example, day and night, cold and hot, female and male, passivity and activity, and the like (for more discussion, see Lozano, 2014a). Fundamental to the *Yinyang* theory is the interdependence between the two opposites when explaining the universe. The theory believes that all manifestations of the universe involve a specific balance between these two opposites. Thus, *yin* increases when *yang* declines (Cheng, 2000). Applied to medicine, *yin* relates to the material aspects of the organism, and *yang* refers to the functions (Tang et al., 2008). TCM holds the belief that any human disease is caused by an imbalance of *yin* and *yang*, and as such, it aims to correct such an imbalance (Chen & Xu, 2003). For instance, a hot symptom will be treated by a drug (in TCM: herbs) with a cold property and vice versa. While the importance of *yin-yang* balance manifests in many aspects, central here is its relationship with qi (energy) and blood. In TCM, qi refers to 'the vital force or energy which flows through a system of channels and conduits in the body, much like the earth's magnetic field', and gives people the capacity to move and work (Chen & Xu, 2003, p. 226). In TCM, the stagnation and deficiency of qi can cause physical disorders.

Also essential in TCM is the Five Phase theory, which describes 'the relationship between the human body and the external environment and the physiological and pathological interactions among the internal organs within the body' (Lao, 1999, p. 218). The theory considers the universe as consisting of five primal elements in an orderly sequence of engendering (Lozano, 2014a): wood, fire, earth, metal, and water. These five elements can explain diverse changes in the universe (for more discussion, see Lao, 1999). The five elements are also used to define the pulse (Matuk, 2006) – a fundamental health indicator in TCM. Similarly, the human body is divided into five functional systems: heart, liver, spleen, lung, and kidney, which govern normal human activities by regulating qi and blood (Chen & Xu, 2003). TCM treats the human body as a holistic unity, and as such, the dysfunction of any part can be explained by a dishar-mony of the body as a whole with the external environment. In TCM path-ology, disease-causing factors include various factors ranging from emotions to a disorderly lifestyle to climate change, and TCM aims to restore harmony. The inexplicability of the TCM foundations, plus the lack of relevant publications in languages other than Chinese, has caused skepticism and criticism about TCM regarding its safety and effectiveness (Tang et al., 2008). However, while lacking scientific foundations, these theories have guided TCM diagnosis and treatment for more than two centuries.

Influenced by these other theories and beliefs, TCM uses a unique diagnostic system that is barely intelligible to WM practitioners. Lozano (2014b, p. 47) describes the TCM diagnostic system as a 'black box' that can be viewed in terms of its outputs (e.g., symptoms, pulse rates) without any knowledge of its internal workings. This unique diagnostic system is called pattern discrimination (Lozano, 2014b) or syndrome differentiation (Hu et al., 2019; Lu et al., 2004), and is pertinent to multiple variables such as patients' lifestyles, constitution, and age. Therefore, TCM is also understood as a personalized medical treatment (Wang & Zhang, 2017). People with various diseases may be treated in the same way if they demonstrate the same pattern or syndrome. Eight patterns are documented and conventionally used to describe diseases: exterior/interior, yin/yang, cold/heat, deficiency/excess (Tang et al., 2008). The diagnosis relies on four examination approaches, namely inspection (e.g., observing the tongue and face), auscultation and olfaction (e.g., evaluating the vocal quality and the odors of breath), inquiry (i.e., information collected from all related areas), and palpation (e.g., examining the pulse) (see Lao, 1999 for more discussion).

To restore harmony, TCM uses several modalities, including Chinese herbal medicine, acupuncture, food and/or diet therapies (for their differences, see Wu & Liang, 2018), Chinese massage, and mind/body exercises. Herbal medi-cine includes plants, minerals, and animal products, which are categorized according to their functions, nature (cool, cold, neutral, hot, and warm), flavor, and temperature (cold and warm) (Lao et al., 2012). These properties correlate with the yin-yang theory as well. According to Zhang (2020), Chinese herbal medicines can be roughly and broadly divided into three types in relation to their effects: clearing heat, eliminating dampness, and detoxifying When treating patients, herbs are usually combined into a homeopathic prescription called a 'medicinal formula' (Xue & O'Brien, 2003, p. 23), consisting of various herbs with separate but complementary functions (see Scheid et al., 2009 for different formulas). The combination of various herbs into a homeopathic prescription is considered to have a 'butterfly effect' (Sheridan et al., 2015, p. S64), whereby each herb lends its minor effects and together they constitute a final product with significant therapeutic efficacy. As Sheridan et al. describe, the homeopathic prescription is decocted in delicate ways to allow the physicochemical interactions of various herbal constituents. Lifestyle is another concept central in the treatment of TCM. As *The Inner Classic of the Yellow Emperor* documents, the secrets for people in China's old days to remain healthy include a balanced diet, a regular bedtime, and effective stress management (Lao, 1999).

1.2.2 Integrating TCM and WM: medical dualism in China

Despite its roots in Chinese history, TCM was challenged by WM in the nineteenth century when several medical missionaries sailed to China to introduce WM. WM quickly dominated the market given its effects in surgery and public health (Xu & Yang, 2009), areas which had not been well developed in China (Tang et al., 2008). We want to underline here that WM has been modified significantly to fit the local practice since its introduction to China (see more discussion in Hsü, 1992).

Since 1949, with the governmental support for developing TCM, an integrated medicine (combining both TCM and WM) accessible to the entire population has become the cornerstone in the health system throughout the nation (Zou, 2016). The campaign to integrate TCM and WM has invoked a national standardization of TCM, ranging from its theoretical foundations to terminology and through to diagnosis and prognosis. Many TCM-specialized hospitals, laboratories, and research teams have been established to promote the standard development of TCM in China (Wang et al., 2016). The campaign allows the integration of knowledge, for example, a mixed treatment of diseases and a joint provision of two clinical practices in the same hospital (Taylor, 2004). Interdisciplinary communication is also encouraged between TCM and WM in education (e.g., curriculum design) and practice. With this kind of integration, patients are able to receive the laboratory tests (e.g., blood tests and X-rays) of WM in addition to TCM herbal therapies (Gu, 1999). As Scheid (2002) notes, patients in China can seek medical assistance from practitioners of both TCM and WM. According to Xu and Chen (2008), over 90% of the Chinese population have sought TCM in their lifetimes. The trend toward using TCM as an alternative healing option is also observed in Western industrialized societies (Taylor, 2004).

Most importantly, the two medical approaches seem to work well by complementing each other in areas where one approach does not help disease management. For example, in chronic care and prevention, TCM is often used as an alternative approach and has been widely applied in many cultures (Fan et al., 2018; Liew et al., 2019; Tsai et al., 2017; Yamada et al., 2016). In the World Health Organization's (WHO's) *International Classification of Diseases 11th Revision (ICD-11)*, TCM is, for the first time, included in this organization's global medical compendium (Cyranoski, 2018). In the present COVID-19 outbreak, early TCM intervention has been reported effective in symptom relief and health recovery (Ren et al., 2020; Zhang, 2020). It seems that the hidden knowledge of TCM is gradually becoming known (though it might not be wholly understood as such) among WM practitioners and laypeople. Given this growing trend of medical integration, examination of the communication practices in both types of interviews is thus necessary. While the subject of communication in medicine has brought about the close collaboration between linguists, communication scholars, and practitioners, most of the existing efforts are fielded in WM with insufficient knowledge about other medical practices that coexist in the broader field of healthcare. As Kim (2014, pp. 520) sensibly reminds us, this dearth of study on complementary and alternative medicines leaves us ignorant of doctor–patient communication in 'professionalized heterodox medical systems'. This is particularly the case for TCM with its philosophical and pathological positions in a myth of theories that are not evidence based. As Taylor (2004, p. 94) points out, 'there remains in today's society this mysterious allure of the Orient and the sacred knowledge contained therein'.

1.3 Organization of the book

The primary aim of this book is to investigate the similarities and differences between TCM and WM (WM practiced in China) in doctor–patient communication. It is closely followed by the secondary aim of suggesting how aspects of differences are attributable to the clinical culture.

A brief outline of the chapters follows. Chapter 2 reviews the rich landscape associated with health communication and applied linguistics. I first describe two types of doctor–patient communication: doctor-centric and patient-centered. I then characterize the nature of doctor-older patient communication. Based on the reviews of earlier studies in doctor–patient communication, I proposed two specific critiques on knowledge about doctor–patient communication, making a case for the present research. In the second half of this chapter, I first introduce the data sources and transcription conventions. I then explain the analytical approaches used for the analysis. The combination of different approaches aims to provide, first, a top-down analysis to generalize the communication patterns and all the components. Based on the big picture, I then use a bottom-up approach to examine the dynamics of interaction.

Chapter 3 examines participants' verbal communication behaviors in medical interactions using the Roter Interaction Analysis System (RIAS). It begins by briefly introducing the coding conventions, presented with examples. Next, the chapter reports the reliability and content validity of the codes in Chinese. Analytical procedures are explained in mathematical formulae. I then report the results and discuss the similarities and differences between TCM and WM in relation to participants' communication styles, presenting a big picture and all its components of the story.

Chapter 4 examines patient's evaluation of their doctors' communication performance across six domains of relational communication. The chapter begins by briefly reviewing factors that affect patient satisfaction. Then I introduce the instrument used to collect patient opinions, describing each of the six domains.

The chapter presents the associations between patients' evaluation of their doctors' communication and global satisfaction with the medical encounter. Additional to the survey findings, this chapter also presents patient comments on their doctors' communication behaviors. The results reported in this chapter extend the RIAS findings. They together constitute the basis for a more rigorous discursive analysis of particular interactional activities that are noted to be different and significant in TCM and WM conversations.

Based on the findings of Chapters 3 and 4, Chapters 5–7 extend these observations by examining the interactional organizations of three activities: diagnostic test recommendation in WM encounters, lifestyle advice-giving and reception in TCM encounters, and nonmedical small talk in both TCM and WM. The activities examined in Chapters 5 and 6 (diagnostic test recommendation and lifestyle advice-giving and reception) constitute, respectively, critical resources for diagnosis and treatment in different encounters. The analyses are primarily Conversation Analysis-driven, focusing on the sequential environments of these activities. The analyses aim to understand where these activities occur in the here-and-now interaction, why in such places, and what functions they serve given their sequential locations. Chapters 5–7 use a bottom-up approach to examine the dynamics of interaction and how participants employ different language resources to collaborate on different projects.

Chapter 8 concludes the book with (i) a revisit of the research design and objectives, (ii) a synthesized summary of the major findings, and (iii) implications and suggestions of future directions that capitalize on the present findings, both for communication scholars and health practitioners.

References

Anderson, G. H. (2006). Peter Parker and the introduction of Western medicine in China. *Mission Studies, 23*(2), 203–238. https://doi.org/10.1163/157338306778985776

Cai, J. F. (1988). Integration of traditional Chinese medicine and Western medicine – right or wrong? *Social Science & Medicine, 27*(5), 521–529. https://doi.org/10.1016/0277-9536(88)90376-0

Chen, K. J., & Xu, H. (2003). The integration of traditional Chinese medicine and Western medicine. *European Review, 11*(2), 225–235. https://doi.org/10.1017/S10627 9870300022X

Cheng, J. T. (2000). Review: Drug therapy in Chinese traditional medicine. *The Journal of Clinical Pharmacology, 40*(5), 445–450. https://doi.org/10.1177/009127000 22009198

Cyranoski, D. (2018). Why Chinese medicine is heading for clinics around the world. *Nature, 561*, 448–450. https://doi.org/10.1038/d41586-018-06782-7

Fan, X., Meng, F., Wang, D., Guo, Q., Ji, Z., Yang, L., & Ogihara, A. (2018). Perceptions of traditional Chinese medicine for chronic disease care and prevention: A cross-sectional study of Chinese hospital-based health care professionals. *BMC Complementary and Alternative Medicine, 18*, 209. https://doi.org/10.1186/s12906-018-2273-y

Gu, Y. G. (1999). A brief introduction to the Chinese health care system. *Health Communication, 11*(3), 203–208. https://doi.org/10.1207/S15327027HC110302

Hesketh, T., & Zhu, W. X. (1997). Health in China: Traditional Chinese medicine: One country, two systems. *BMJ*, *315*, 115–117. https://doi.org/10.1136/bmj. 315.7100.115

Hsü, E. (1992). The reception of Western medicine in China: Examples from Yunnan. In P. Petitjean, C. Jami, & A. M. Moulin (Eds.), *Science and empires: Historical studies about scientific development and European expansion* (pp. 89–101). Dordrecht: Springer. https://doi.org/10.1007/978-94-011-2594-9_11

Hu, Q., Yu, T., Li, J., Yu, Q., Zhu, L., & Gu, Y. (2019). End-to-End syndrome differentiation of Yin deficiency and Yang deficiency in traditional Chinese medicine. *Computer Methods and Programs in Biomedicine*, *174*, 9–15. https://doi.org/10.1016/j. cmpb.2018.10.011

Kim, K. (2014). Negotiation of health, illness, and treatment in Korean oriental medical discourse. In H. E. Hamilton & W-y. S. Chou (Eds.), *The Routledge handbook of language and health communication* (pp. 520–538). Abingdon: Routledge.

Kong, Y. C. (2010). *Huangdi Neijing: A synopsis with commentaries.* Hong Kong: The Chinese University of Hong Kong Press. https://doi.org/10.2307/j.ctt1p9wqh4

Lao, L. X. (1999). Traditional Chinese medicine. In W. B. Jonas & J. S. Levin (Eds.), *Essentials of complementary and alternative medicine* (pp. 216–232). Baltimore: Lippincott Williams & Wilkins.

Lao, L. X., Xu, L., & Xu, S. F. (2012). Traditional Chinese medicine. In A. Längler, P. J. Mansky, & G. Seifert (Eds.), *Integrative pediatric oncology* (pp. 125–135). New York: Springer. https://doi.org/10.1007/978-3-642-04201-0_9

Liew, A. C., Peh, K-K., Tan, B. S., Zhao, W., & Tangiisuran, B. (2019). Evaluation of chemotherapy-induced toxicity and health-related quality of life amongst early-stage breast cancer patients receiving Chinese herbal medicine in Malaysia. *Supportive Care in Cancer*, *27*, 4515–4524. https://doi.org/10.1007/s00520-019-04724-1

Lozano, F. (2014a). Basic theories of traditional Chinese medicine. In Y. C. Lin & E. S. Z. Hsu (Eds.), *Acupuncture for pain management* (pp. 13–43). London & New York: Springer. https://doi.org/10.1007/978-1-4614-5275-1_2

Lozano, F. (2014b). Pattern discrimination in traditional Chinese medicine (TCM). In Y. C. Lin & E. S. Z. Hsu (Eds.), *Acupuncture for pain management* (pp. 45–72). London & New York: Springer. https://doi.org/10.1007/978-1-4614-5275-1_3

Lu, A. P., Jia, H. W., Xiao, C., & Lu, Q. P. (2004). Theory of traditional Chinese and medicine and therapeutic method of diseases. *World Journal of Gastroenterology*, *10*(13), 1854–1856. https://doi.org/10.3748/wjg.v10.i13.1854

Matuk, C. (2006). Seeing the body: The divergence of ancient Chinese and western medical illustration. *Journal of Biocommunication*, *32*(1), 8.

Reading, A. (1977). Illness and disease. *Medical Clinics of North America*, *61*(4), 703–710. https://doi.org/10.1007/978-1-4614-5275-1_2

Ren, J. L., Zhang, A. H., & Wang, X. J. (2020). Traditional Chinese medicine for COVID-19 treatment. *Pharmacological Research*, *155*, 104743. https://doi.org/10.1016/j.phrs.2020.104743

Scheid, V. (2002). *Chinese medicine in contemporary China: Plurality and synthesis.* Durham & London: Duke University Press. https://doi.org/10.1215/9780822383710

Scheid, V., Bensky, D., Ellis, A., & Barolet, R. (2009). *Chinese herbal medicine: Formulas and strategies.* Seattle: Eastland Press.

Sheridan, H., Kopp, B., Krenn, L., Guo, D., & Sendker, J. (2015). Traditional Chinese herbal medicine preparation: Invoking the butterfly effect. *Science*, *350*(6263): S64–S66.

Street, R. L. Jr. (2013). How clinician–patient communication contributes to health improvement: Modeling pathways from talk to outcome. *Patient Education and Counseling*, *92*(3), 286–291. https://doi.org/10.1016/j.pec.2013.05.004

Tang, J. L., Liu, B. Y., & Ma, K. W. (2008). Traditional Chinese medicine. *The Lancet*, *372*(9654), 1938–1940. https://doi.org/10.1016/S0140-6736(08)61354-9

Taylor, K. (2004). Divergent interests and cultivated misunderstandings: The influence of the West on modern Chinese medicine. *Social History of Medicine*, *17*(1), 93–111. https://doi.org/10.1093/shm/17.1.93

Tsai, T-Y., Livneh, H., Hung, T-H., Lin, I-H., Lu, M-C., & Yeh, C-C. (2017). Associations between prescribed Chinese herbal medicine and risk of hepatocellular carcinoma in patients with chronic hepatitis B: a nationwide population-based cohort study. *BMJ Open*, *7*, e014571. http://dx.doi.org/10.1136/bmjopen-2016-014571

Wang, J., Guo, Y., & Li, L. (2016). Current status of standardization of traditional Chinese medicine in China. *Evidence-Based Complementary and Alternative Medicine*, 2016, 9123103. https://doi.org/10.1155/2016/9123103

Wang, W-J. & Zhang, T. (2017). Integration of traditional Chinese medicine and Western medicine in the era of precision medicine. *Journal of Integrative Medicine*, *15*(1), 1–7. https://doi.org/10.1016/S2095-4964(17)60314-5

Williams, S., Weinman, J., & Dale, J. (1998). Doctor–patient communication and patient satisfaction: A review. *Family Practice*, *15*(5), 480–492. https://psycnet.apa.org/doi/10.1093/fampra/15.5.480

Wu, Q., & Liang, X. (2018). Food therapy and medical diet therapy of traditional Chinese medicine. *Clinical Nutrition Experimental*, *18*, 1–5. https://doi.org/10.1016/j.yclnex.2018.01.001

Xu, H., & Chen, K. (2008). Integrative medicine: The experience from China. *The Journal of Alternative and Complementary Medicine*, *14*(1), 3–7. https://doi.org/10.1089/acm.2006.6329

Xu, J., & Yang, Y. (2009). Traditional Chinese medicine in the Chinese health care system. *Health Policy*, *90*(2–3): 133–139. https://doi.org/10.1016/j.healthpol.2008.09.003

Xue, C. C., & O'Brien, K. A. (2003). Modalities of Chinese medicine. In P. C. Leung, C. C. Xue, & Y. C. Cheng (Eds.), *A comprehensive guide to Chinese medicine* (pp. 19–46). Hackensack, NJ: World Scientific. https://doi.org/10.1142/9789812794987_0002

Yamada, T., Wajima, T., Nakaminami, H., Kobayashi, K., Ikoshi, H., & Noguchi, N. (2016). The modified Gingyo-san, a Chinese herbal medicine, has direct antibacterial effects against respiratory pathogens. *BMC Complementary and Alternative Medicine*, *16*, 463. https://doi.org/10.1186/s12906-016-1431-3

Zhang, K. (2020). Is traditional Chinese medicine useful in the treatment of COVID-19?. *American Journal of Emergency Medicine*, *38*(10), P2238. https://doi.org/10.1016/j.ajem.2020.03.046

Zou, P. (2016). Traditional Chinese medicine, food therapy, and hypertension control: A narrative review of Chinese literature. *American Journal of Chinese Medicine*, *44*(8), 1579–1594. https://doi.org/10.1142/S0192415X16500889

2 Preliminaries and methodology

2.1 Doctor–older patient communication and patient satisfaction

2.1.1 From doctor-centric to patient-centered

In the last few decades, concern for provider-patient talk has been fueled by a growing awareness of the significance of talk in medical encounters. Much of the earlier knowledge in this field is coming out of the United States and some European countries where WM is the dominant health provider. One of the pioneering efforts in explaining doctor–patient relationships is that offered by American sociologist Talcott Parsons. He proposed the 'sick role' concept and considered illness a form of social deviance (Parsons, 1951). Parsons considered the sick role as an essential mechanism of social control. From a Parsonian perspective, the state of being sick is undesirable and is beyond personal control (Parsons, 1975). While being temporarily exempted from ordinary social obligations and expectations, the sick person has no autonomy in their treatment and is therefore dependent on the health agent for an early health recovery (Varul, 2010). In other words, conventional medical interactions feature a paternalistic relationship between the provider and the patient. For many decades, such paternalism was a common feature of provider-patient interactions in many cultures, particularly the United States.

Despite its influence, Parson's sick-role concept was critiqued and later abandoned by sociologists (see Burnham, 2014 for a review). One of the criticisms against it relates to its focus on acute care with insufficient embrace of chronic and preventive care (Parsons, 1975). This new wave in chronic care is probably fueled by the rise of chronic conditions over the past few decades. Unlike the acutely ill person, the chronically ill person navigates between being sick and being normal like other individuals who are able to participate in their everyday social obligations. Radley (2004, p. 139) metaphorically described the chronically ill as 'living with illness in a world of health'. From the 1970s onward, with the growth in medical care for chronic illness, there has been a shift in discussion of patient behavior from sick to healthy. As Varul (2010, p. 72) sensibly reminded us, the sick role concept is problematic and obsolete with the rise of chronic diseases and 'the pathologization of everyday behaviors in health promotion'.

DOI: 10.4324/9781003161929-2

This thrust for health promotion has fueled a change in the provider-patient relationship from provider-centric to patient- or person-centered. High levels of patient-centeredness are associated with better medical outcomes such as greater satisfaction, better doctor–patient relationship, and improved treatment outcomes (Carrard et al., 2018; Plewnia et al., 2016; Saha & Beach, 2011). Interestingly, the anticipated outcomes of providing patient-centered care (PCC) are in accord with the three functions of medical interviews: building an effective provider-patient relationship, understanding and assessing patient problems, and collaborating on problem management (Cole & Bird, 2013).

Despite the extensive studies on patient-centeredness and its effectiveness on medical outcomes, there is little uniformity in the literature on how patient-centeredness is defined (e.g., Mead & Bower, 2000; Little et al., 2001). Hobbs (2009) contended that it is a poorly conceptualized phenomenon. Stewart (2001) argued that central to providing PCC is to take into account the individual needs of the patient (e.g., information needs, emotional needs, and decision-making preferences), to explore their main reason for the visit and their primary concerns, to understand different aspects of their world, to seek health prevention and promotion, and to enhance the continuing provider-patient relationship (see also Stewart et al., 2003). Building on Stewart et al.'s (2003) model of PCC, Hudon et al. (2012) explored this concept in chronic disease management. They examined the findings of earlier research work published from 1980 to 2009. Six major themes are addressed. Some of the themes nicely correspond to Stewart et al.'s model. For example, the theme 'starting from the patient's situation' involves exploring patients' disease (e.g., by history and diagnostic tests) and illness (e.g., feelings about being ill, patients' self-explanations, impacts on life, and patient expectations) (see Brown et al., 1999 for the conceptual differences) and understanding the patient as a whole person (i.e., focusing not only on patients' biomedical concerns but also their lifeworlds). This last dimension of attending to the patient as an entire person seems to be universally agreed upon by existing definitions of PCC.

Hudon et al. (2012) observed three new themes related to PCC: legitimizing the illness experience, offering realistic hope, and providing advocacy for the patient in the healthcare system. According to these scholars, all the themes reviewed include a longitudinal dimension by considering patients' needs and wants over time along the trajectory of illness. Hudon et al.'s thematic analysis has advanced the understanding of PCC in chronic care encounters. Similarly, Brickley et al. (2021) synthesized findings on PCC in general practitioner (GP) practice and proposed a model with four major PCC components. Their model gives considerable weight to the theme of 'experiencing time' with two subdimensions: the length of the encounter and a longitudinal GP-patient relationship. According to Brickley et al., this theme relates closely to the rest of the PCC components because it ensures the accomplishment of all institutional and interactional tasks. For example, the length of the encounter may readily account for the extent to which the GP attends to the patient and explores their personal life to understand the patient as a whole person. Despite the diversity in how PCC is defined, most of the earlier work seems to agree that effective PCC encounters should consider the varying needs of patients (in terms of disease, biomedical and psychosocial issues, medical experience and personal life), orient to the continuity of care and relationship, and seek common ground and goals.

Extensive studies have reported strong associations between PCC and older patient outcomes (e.g., Finkelstein et al., 2017; Liang et al., 2006). Phillips et al. (2012) examined the association between patient satisfaction and patients' perceived interpersonal sensitivity of the provider (i.e., patient trust, feelings that providers treat them with respect and dignity, and feelings about shared understanding). Their data are drawn from a nationwide survey of the population in the United States. Among the 2,075 patients aged more than 50 years, they report strong associations between patients' perceived interpersonal sensitivity and satisfaction with medical care. Most importantly, while their data include people of various ethnic and racial backgrounds, the association between the two variables is persistent among all ethnic and racial groups. This strong need for interpersonal care is more explicitly reflected in Marcinowicz et al.'s (2014) interviews with Polish older patients aged 65 and above. According to Marcinowicz et al. (2014), while older patients assess physician behaviors on both task performance (e.g., giving information and questioning) and affective domains of communication, they pay more attention to the affective behaviors. In their study, physician behaviors fielded into the affective domain include social conversation, understanding (e.g., showing empathy, attentive listening, and showing interest), providing support, indicating friendliness, allowing sufficient consultation time for the patient to raise their concerns, and partnership building (e.g., joint decision-making). These affective behaviors demonstrate physicians' patient-centric views, which are expected and positively evaluated by older patients. Marcinowicz et al. also point out that older patients are particularly attentive to physician behaviors that index friendliness, such as joking and social conversation. As Baker et al. (2020) indicated, patients want both emotional and medical needs met in a balanced way to allow both interpersonal and intergroup communication. This is particularly so for older patients with multiple chronic conditions associated with aging. To these patients, regular visits may occur to address various health-related issues such as a physical checkup, medication refills, and other aspects of chronic disease management. Thus, communication featuring PCC may stand as an important source of biomedical and interpersonal care.

2.1.2 *Features of doctor-older patient communication*

Unlike doctor-younger patient communication, communication with older patients is more complicated for several reasons. For example, due to age-related physiological impairments, older patients can be slow or less effective in presenting their concerns and necessary information for diagnosis. Moreover, older patients typically see their doctors with a combination of physiological and psychological problems that add uncertainties to the diagnosis and treatment. As

Adelman, Greene, and Charon (1991) stated, there are unique features in doctor-older patient communication. Research on this population group deserves subjective investigation rather than examining them as a subgroup of a population.

One of the earlier studies examining issues in provider-elderly patient interactions is Haug and Ory (1987). Their review discussed various factors such as provider and patient characteristics, contextual and situational factors, and interactional asymmetry that might affect the outcome of the interaction. Haug and Ory seem to take a negative view of the 'aged' role. They considered aging as a 'deficit' (p. 10) for care and interactions. For example, they pointed out that since elderly patients are slow in reacting, they might take longer to present necessary information for diagnosis and treatment, causing annoyance to their providers, particularly to doctors with a busy schedule. Haug and Ory also summarized, from extant studies, that when communicating with elderly patients, doctors tend to take a detached stance by various means such as withholding information. Their review provides the groundwork for more recent studies focusing on the impact of age on interaction.

One feature of doctor-older patient encounters is the lack of concordance in information needs or topics of interest between doctors and patients. In a seminal publication, Mishler (1984) described a discrepancy between doctor and patient agendas: while doctors give primacy to a medical agenda by concentrating on the assessment and treatment of medication-related problems, patients sometimes pursue a lifeworld agenda by discussing their psychosocial concerns and other issues they experience in everyday life. This discrepancy is particularly noted in older patient encounters, as aging usually relates to psychological health (Mitina et al., 2020). According to Greene and Adelman (1996), the basic tenet of geriatric medicine is to attend to the patients' biomedical and psychosocial concerns for proper diagnosis and treatment. However, studies have indicated infrequent discussions on psychosocial-related topics in medical encounters due to various factors such as patient reluctance, doctors' agist bias, and situational factors like insufficient time (see Greene & Adelman, 1996 for a review). Greene et al. (1989) found that the level of concordance in topics discussed is significantly lower in older patient visits than in younger patient visits. Likewise, Adelman et al. (1991) summarized from their review of the literature that while older patients are more likely to raise psychosocial topics than younger adults, doctors are more attentive to medical problems and less to psychosocial discussions with their older patients than with younger patients. This lack of concordance or provider-patient agreement in primary care encounters seems to be consistently reported in the literature (Maly et al., 2002; Schumacher et al., 2013). Recent studies, particularly those in oncological settings, have also observed such informational disconcordance, focusing mainly on older patients' unmet informational needs (Goldfarb & Casillas, 2014; van Weert et al., 2013; Wu et al., 2020). Yet, other studies also suggest that this information discrepancy is sometimes supported by the companion of the patient (Daher, 2012), particularly in some Asian cultures like China (Gan et al., 2017; Tse et al., 2013; Yi et al., 2016). In a recent study of cancer diagnosis disclosure, Liu et al. (2018) found that of the 124 pairs of patients and families in a Chinese tertiary hospital, more than 60% of the patients did not know their diagnosis before chemotherapy, and that more patients than family members wanted the patients to be informed about a diagnosis.

Another level of disconcordance lies in the values and goals for care, which are generally reported as poor among patients with multiple chronic conditions (Kuluski et al., 2019). In a study of older multimorbid patients (mean age 65) with a life-threatening disease, Naik et al. (2016) observed five core values that patients consider primary, namely self-sufficiency, life enjoyment, connectedness and legacy (e.g., healthy social and spiritual relationships), balancing quality and length of time, and engagement in care. Studies have agreed that patients with multimorbidity prioritize fixing symptoms and functional challenges, maintaining emotional and behavioral health, and staying safe (Kuluski et al., 2013, 2019). Vermunt et al. (2017) examined the goals of health providers, including disease or symptom-specific goals, functional goals, and fundamental goals. They defined disease or symptom-specific goals as those relating to medical diagnosis and treatment, whereas functional goals were those about fixing functional health. The third type – the fundamental goals – covers a broad spectrum of patients' life properties, broadly reflecting their views about the future of their life. Vermunt et al. observed variation in providers' consideration of fundamental goals, with no consideration, implicit consideration, and explicit consideration orientations. In other words, while all health providers are aware of patients' need for fixing symptoms and functional challenges, consideration of patients' life properties is not a universal practice.

Concordance between the professional and the patient requires communication regarding patients' priorities so that patient preference and professional experience can nicely merge to work out the best treatment. This process is known as shared decision-making. Recent studies have suggested the importance of shared decision-making in treating older multimorbid patients (Hoffmann et al., 2018). However, shared decision-making is complicated when treating older multimorbid patients, as the treatment is not the sum of the parts, and the decision-making process is likely to be more complicated with the involvement of the patient's family. Therefore, good communication is required between health providers and patients and their families as regards the patient's primary concerns, priorities, preferences, short- and long-term goals, and treatment options. Previous studies also indicate that preference for shared decision-making declines with aging (Arora & McHorney, 2000; Schulman-Green et al., 2006). Compared with other factors, shared decision-making can be less of a concern to older patients. For example, Greene et al. (1994) found that elderly (no less than 60 years old) patients' satisfaction is positively associated with factors such as the length of the visit, shared laughter, and the doctors' attentiveness to patient-initiated topics. They also observed that egalitarian and joint decision-making might be less of a concern to older patients than other interactional features such as doctors' attentiveness to patient affect. Such deference to doctors among older patients in decision-making is widely reported in the literature (Stewart et al., 2000; Levinson et al., 2005). In a study of decision control preferences among diverse older adults in the United States, Chiu et al. (2016) found that nearly one-fifth of adults wanted their doctors to make medical decisions for them.

Older patients' passivity toward engaging in shared decision-making is even greater with an increasing number of chronic conditions (Belcher et al., 2005; Chi et al., 2017). In the latest review, Pel-Little et al. (2021) discussed the barriers and facilitators for shared decision-making between professionals and their older patients with chronic conditions. Their findings suggest that apart from health-related issues such as cognitive and physical impairment, other inter-actional factors like lack of empathy and underevaluation of patients' expertise might affect patients' confidence in contributing to the shared decision-making. However, understanding the patient's values, recognizing the patient's expertise, and asking questions about their main worries could facilitate patients' involve-ment in decision-making. Pel-Little et al.'s review thus points to the importance of PCC in treating older patients with chronic conditions.

2.2 A critique of current studies in doctor-older patient communication

2.2.1 Insufficient understanding of medical interactions in regular chronic visits

As Haug and Ory (1987) stated, a routine checkup for a chronic condition can engender a significantly different interaction than would occur if a patient visits for a new life-threatening disease. While most of the earlier work in the field of health communication focuses on acute care visits (see Barnes, 2019), less is known about the situation in regular chronic visits. Yet, given the prominence of chronic diseases in the current society, examining these encounters is critical. On the one hand, a chronic encounter usually features a progression of treatment. Patients with chronic conditions are more likely than those with acute conditions to visit the same doctor for routine checkups. In that sense, the patient and the doctor know each other better than they would if the patient were a first-time visitor. Therefore, a continuity of cure and care is possible in regular chronic encounters. Thus, examining such encounters can help us better understand issues such as the doctor–patient relationship and its association with patient outcomes. On the other hand, given the various age-related diseases and illnesses, chronic encounters are richer sources of doctor-older patient interactions than acute visits and are subject to closer investigations.

2.2.2 Insufficient understanding of medical interactions in TCM and WM

Despite the extensive research on doctor–patient communication and patient sat-isfaction in the literature, most of the existing research is situated in WM in the United States, the United Kingdom, and some European countries. Little is said about other medical practices that also exist in the broader healthcare market. Given the trend of medical dualism or pluralism, exploring the clinical differences with regard to participants' communicative styles and language representations is necessary. Such knowledge can help us better understand the tie between communication, clinical culture, and patient outcomes.

One of the few exceptions among studies that investigate participants' language features in TCM is Gu (1996), which examined how doctors and patients attain their goals while building interpersonal relations through the interaction. Gu's observation of medical interactions in both WM and TCM as a 'goal-directed discourse' (1996, p. 157) supports the conventional understanding of medical encounters as task oriented. For instance, Gu noted that medical interactions may start without a greeting between the two participants. Such 'greetingless discourse' (Gu, 1996, p. 169) is sometimes replaced by the doctor's paralinguistic cues like pointing to the seat or a strictly task-oriented inquiry into the patient's major concerns. Lack of small talk is another observation in Gu's study, adding support to his observation of medical interactions in China as goal directed. Regarding the clinical differences, Gu found that TCM features a goal-attaining journey different from the WM routines. Specifically, Gu identified unique TCM phases, including *jiezhen* (taking a consultation), *zhenduan* (diagnosis), *lifa* (treatment decision-making), *chufang* (prescribing), and *tiaoli* (recuperation). The last of the five phases involves communication on diet restrictions and recommendations. Gu argued that one remarkable difference between TCM and WM is that while TCM interactions usually end with recuperative advice, such action is rare in WM encounters. Another marked difference is the rarity of continuity of care in WM. According to Gu, patients who see TCM doctors are usually encouraged to visit the same doctor until they are cured. While Gu's study provides a general description of the communication features in both TCM and WM, these features were not subject to comprehensive analysis.

Chung et al. (2009) examined public evaluations of medical consultations in both Western and traditional Chinese clinics in Hong Kong. Data were collected from a household survey conducted by the Census and Statistics Department of the Local Government. People who were at least 15 years old and had received outpatient care within the past 30 days were considered eligible. Questionnaires were designed to collect people's evaluations of their doctors regarding four interactional behaviors, namely attentive listening, information explanation, showing respect, and consultation length. Their findings indicate a marked difference between TCM and WM: while WM patients were dissatisfied with all aspects of the survey items (listening, explanation, respect, time allocation, and global assessment), TCM patients expressed greater satisfaction with their doctors in terms of listening skills.

Similar findings were reported in Wang (2010) in a comparative study between China and the United States. The findings are based on 26 in-depth interviews and 2,377 surveys (1,097 Chinese and 1,287 Americans). Wang argueg that TCM doctors are better communicators than WM doctors. According to Wang, communication plays an essential part in doctor–patient interactions, given the unique diagnostic approach in TCM. Like Gu (1996), Wang also reported a long-term doctor–patient relationship in TCM encounters. Apart from the fact that TCM treatment usually asks for several follow-up visits, Wang also contended that TCM doctors are more accessible. As Wang argued, 'another reason is that western medicine doctors were much busier than traditional Chinese medicine doctors, so they didn't have enough time to [...] follow any specific patients' case' (p. 88). Wang concluded that TCM visits demonstrate better doctor performance in observing, listening, and asking questions. While Wang's study is quite illuminating to the present research in understanding the similarities and differences between TCM and WM concerning doctor–patient communication and patient satisfaction, one critique of his study is that the findings are based on self-reported surveys and interviews. In addition, most of the participants in the study had limited experience with TCM doctors. In that sense, the findings are less informative in the revelation of the TCM interactions in situ. Furthermore, since the WM data in Wang's study is collected in the United States, the differences between TCM and WM reported in Wang's investigation could be a matter of cultural rather than clinical difference.

2.2.3 Extending current research in TCM and WM practiced in China

The present review of research ultimately aims to identify the limitations of doctor–patient communication and patient satisfaction to advance our theoretical and context-based understanding of doctor–patient communication and patient satisfaction in different clinical practices that coexist in the healthcare market.

This research provides both a 'top-down' and a 'bottom-up' examination of doctor–patient interactions and patient satisfaction in chronic settings in TCM and WM practiced in China. For the top-down investigation, participants' communication behaviors are examined using the Roter Interaction Analysis System (Roter, 1977), one of the widely used interaction analysis approaches in the field. Patient evaluations are collected using the Relational Communication Scale (Burgoon et al., 1987). For the bottom-up investigation, Conversation Analysis (CA) and frame analysis are used to examine the micro language features that differentiate TCM and WM in relation to communication styles.

The primary research objective is to explore the similarities and differences between TCM and WM in relation to doctor–patient communication and the impact on patient satisfaction. Three interdependent yet methodologically diverse studies will be conducted to: (i) Explore the clinical similarities and differences in relation to participants' communication behaviors during medical consultations; (ii) Examine patient evaluations of doctors' communication styles and whether these evaluations correlate to global patient satisfaction; and (iii) Investigate specific activities/actions that differentiate TCM and WM regarding doctor–patient communication.

2.3 Data sources and transcription conventions

Hospitals in China are classified into three levels in ascending order, and each level is subclassified into two grades in descending order. Grade-A-Level-Three hospitals (or Grade-A Tertiary Hospitals, see Fang, 2017) are considered better than others and provide more comprehensive healthcare services. In addition, most of these hospitals offer both TCM and WM healthcare and have an independent dispensary for TCM, WM, and patent medicine. Therefore, these hospitals are usually busier, with a large patient volume (see Hu & Zhang, 2015). For patient variability, this study was carried out in one such hospital (Hospital A).

There is no general practitioner in Chinese hospitals. Patients go directly to the hospital and decide on an outpatient department suitable for them based on their knowledge. The function of the outpatient department is similar to that of the GP (Hougaard et al., 2011). Each outpatient department provides both specialist and non-specialist services. Usually, the specialist has an independent consultation room, while a non-specialist has to share their space with others. To secure privacy, this study only considers patient-specialist consultations.

This study focuses on older adults with chronic conditions. Participants were recruited from the Divisions of Gastroenterology and Internal Traditional Chinese Medicine within Hospital A. The Division of Gastroenterology (WM) was chosen because Gastroenterology, as the key discipline of Hospital A, attracts a considerable number of outpatients and inpatients. Ethical approval was granted by both the Ethical Committee of the hospital and my home university. Six medical specialists and 69 older adults (34 male, 35 female) agreed to participate in this study. Of the six medical specialists, three were from the Division of Gastroenterology and three were from Internal Traditional Chinese Medicine. Patients were approached at the waiting area outside the outpatient department. Patients were considered eligible if they were (1) no less than 50 years old (earliest legitimate age of retirement), (2) formally diagnosed with a clinical report of chronic disease, (3) capable of independent communication with no mental disease, (4) had both TCM and WM consultation experiences, and (5) they had visited the same doctor before. I intentionally excluded initial visits to examine doctor–patient communication in repeat encounters. Informed consent was obtained from all the participants prior to their participation. The average patient age was 63 years (SD = 8.5). All the medical consultations were audio-recorded. The average length of visit was 5.5 min (SD = 1.75) for TCM and 3.0 (SD = 1.8) for WM, $p < 0.01$, $r = 0.6$.

To transcribe the data, I use CA conventions following Jefferson (2004). I provide three-line transcripts where the first line presents the Chinese pinyin original; the second line offers a word-by-word gloss of the Chinese; the third line provides the idiomatic translation. When translating, I try to be faithful and produce the precise contextual meaning of the source language within the constraints of English grammar. In the transcripts, all the particles (e.g., *ma*, *ba*, *ou*, and *de*) are transcribed as PRT and translated as such. In all the data presented in this volume, D stands for the doctor, and P stands for the patient.

2.4 Methodology used for three separate studies

2.4.1 Process/interaction analysis

A commonly used method to handle the interaction data is applying specific process/interaction analysis schemes (also known as observation protocols or coding schemes) through which categorization of different communication behaviors is feasible (Koenig & Robinson, 2014). Studies within this methodological tradition collect authentic recordings (audio or video) of conversational interactions. Transcriptions may or may not be required.

The application of such an approach in healthcare studies was introduced by Barbara Korsch and her associates, whose early studies (Korsch et al., 1968; Korsch & Negrete, 1972) furnish quantifiable evidence for medical interaction exchanges. Using Bales' (1950) Interaction Process Analysis, these scholars coded the content of the interchanges between doctors and patients, providing empirical evidence on the applicability of interaction process analysis to the study of doctor–patient interaction. There exist several coding schemes to describe the dynamics of the medical encounter, such as Bales' (1950) Process Analysis System, Roter's (1977) Interaction Analysis System (RIAS), Stiles' (1981) Verbal Response Mode System, and the Multidimensional Interaction Analysis (MDIA) developed by Adelman, Greene, Charon, and their colleagues in a series of studies (Adelman et al., 1991, 1992, 2000; Charon et al., 1994). These coding schemes are widely applied to the investigation of doctor–patient communication. While the four observational schemes and those not cited here vary in their units of analysis (utterances, interpersonal intent, syntactic unit, and topic), exhaustiveness of the behavior categories, and target participants (care providers, patients, family members), a commonality between them is that they allow a quantitative calculation of qualitative data by classifying different role behaviors.

This research uses RIAS. Determination on coding medical interactions by RIAS is based on its distinction between instrumental and affective behaviors (Roter & Larson, 2002), which gives equal weight to both the biomedical and relational aspects of communication. Derived from social exchange theories concerning interpersonal influence, empowerment, reciprocity, and problem-solving (Ellington et al., 2014; Roter & Larson, 2002), RIAS views the interactional processes of medical consultations as a locus of human activity where resource exchange is realized through provider-patient dialogues (Roter, 2010). It suggests that this kind of dialogue shapes the relationship between care providers and patients and reflects participants' social roles and responsibilities. For instance, the patient's responsibility to account for their symptoms and medical histories should be reciprocated by their care providers informing them well, and vice versa (Roter & Hall, 1991). The notions of exchange and interpersonal influence determine the communication behaviors of the provider and the patient. Grounded in this theoretical orientation, RIAS classifies communication behaviors in medical visits into two domains: instrumental (task-based) and affective (socio-emotional) for both providers and patients. Instrumental behavior is defined as 'technically based skills used in problem-solving, which compose the base of expertness for which the physician is consulted' (Hall et al., 1987, p. 400). Affective behavior is defined as behaviors aimed at building a rapport between physicians and patients (Roter & Larson, 2002), including expression with explicit socio-emotional content (Hall et al., 1987). Patient behaviors are defined in a similar manner. This parallel treatment of both physician and patient behaviors allows interpretation of how the behavior of one party affects the other's response and the building of a therapeutic relationship.

To measure participant communication behaviors, RIAS categorizes the two broad domains into different communication elements and subsequently uses the approach of cluster analysis to provide statistical evidence of the theoretical underpinning of participants' communication patterns. The unit of analysis is the utterance, operationalized as 'the smallest discriminable speech segment to which a coder can assign a classification and which expresses or implies a complete thought' (Roter et al., 1987, p. 440). In RIAS, an utterance is also coded based upon a pause. According to the RIAS manual, a sentence divided by a pause of more than one second would be considered as being composed of two utterances (Sandvik et al., 2002). Therefore an utterance can be as lengthy as a sentence or as short as a single word (e.g., *yeah*). Each utterance is assigned one of the 43 exclusive communication elements, among which 29 are instrumental and 14 are socio-emotional (see Sandvik et al., 2002 for illustration). These categories reflect both the form (i.e., the type of activities) (e.g., questions, information-giving, counseling, giving directions) and the content (lifestyle, medical condition, therapeutic regimen, and others) of the dyadic interaction. By capturing specific verbal behaviors (e.g., questioning on medical condition), RIAS allows for a detailed categorization and analysis of participants' interaction at both the micro (comparison of particular behaviors) and the macro level (comparisons at a broader level). Apart from components that apply to care providers and patients, some elements are either provider-exclusive (e.g., counseling) or patient-exclusive (e.g., request for service). In total, these communication elements capture both cure- and care-oriented behaviors, recognized as the two fundamental needs of the patient (Ong et al., 1995, 1998).

RIAS has shown advantages over other coding systems with regard to its practicality, functionality, adaptability, and flexibility (Roter & Larson, 2002). The reliability and content validity of RIAS has been examined broadly in different clinical settings, including primary care (Roter & Larson, 2001), obstetrics and gynecology (Roter et al., 1999), oncology (Ong et al., 1998), emergency care (Wissow et al., 1998), and pharmaceutical care (Pelicano-Romano et al., 2013), and specific diagnostic categories such as asthma and diabetes (Roter & Larson, 2002). As Heritage and Maynard (2006) commented, RIAS is by far the most influential and widely used coding scheme. Inui et al. (1982) justified the appropriateness, applicability, and explanatory power of RIAS by comparing it with the Bales' approach and the Verbal Response Mode System across 101 clinical visits. These scholars concluded that compared with the two other schemes, RIAS is 'best suited to clinical encounters' (p. 548), possibly because it may be used in capturing different verbal behaviors within the instrumental domain of doctor–patient communication. The flexibility of RIAS as a coding framework lies in its viability for the coder to conduct cluster analysis by grouping behaviors of a similar fashion for an in-depth understanding of the dynamic of medical communication. For example, Ong et al. (1998), in their study of oncological consultations, explored four instrumental clusters (giving information, giving directions, asking questions, and counseling) and four affective clusters (social behavior, verbal attentiveness, showing concern, and negative talk).

Like other interaction analysis approaches, while RIAS is powerful in 'global characterizations of interactional situations' (Peräkylä, 2004, p. 1), it is weak in revealing the 'layers of organization [...] that give structure to interactional situations' (Peräkylä, 2004, p. 1). As Sandvik et al. (2002, p. 235) stated, RIAS is not designed to 'assess what type of answer is typically given to a specific type of question'. In other words, while RIAS can identify a behavior, it cannot tell us why and how the behavior is performed or responded to as such. To answer this question, I use CA and frame analysis.

2.4.2 Evaluating patient satisfaction

To evaluate patient satisfaction, questionnaires are distributed to patients after their medical interviews. As a standard method for data collection, and the most widely used tool in quantitative studies, questionnaires are broadly adopted in social science research. Despite the heterogeneity of questionnaires to evaluate patient satisfaction, most of them are fielded for one of two purposes: (1) to evaluate health professionals' quality of services; and (2) to predict health and illness behaviors on the assumption that variation in patient satisfaction will lead to different behaviors (Ware et al., 1978). This study evaluates professionals' quality of services, focusing on a range of professionals' affective communication behaviors.

The study uses the short form (14-item scale) of the Relational Communication Scale (RCS) (Burgoon & Hale, 1987) to assess patient satisfaction about their medical consultations, focusing primarily on the interactional performance rather than the technical expertise of the doctor. The RCS was developed by reviewing other measurements in prior studies and sifting from them concepts and wording appropriate to relational communication (Burgoon & Hale, 1984, 1987). After several modifications, the initial 32 items were developed into 30 items, fielded into eight dimensions of relational communication (see Burgoon & Hale, 1987). Strong validity and high reliability were reported. Gallagher et al. (2001) claimed that the RCS is 'the only extant instrument developed explicitly to measure the relational communication aspects of the doctor–patient interaction' (p. 212).

Elsewhere, Burgoon et al. (1987) proposed a short form of RCS, which contains only 14 items. Items were fielded into six domains of relational communication: (a) immediacy – the extent to which closeness and distance are expressed, (b) dominance – the degree to which equality and mutuality is demonstrated, (c) formality – the extent to which medical interviews are either formal or informal, (d) receptivity – the extent to which openness is expressed and rapport is shown, (e) composure – whether the participant is anxious or composed, and (f) similarity – the degree to which one feels similar or different in terms of values and attitudes. The applicability of RCS-14 among the Chinese population was reported by Wang (2010) in a cross-cultural study of doctor–patient interactions.

2.4.3 Conversation Analysis

Arising in sociology, CA is one approach within discourse analysis that studies the organization and orderliness of social interaction, using a bottom-up approach to research and theorizing. Inspired by Goffman's (1983) work on interaction order and Garfinkel's (1967) research in ethnomethodology (particularly the notions of shared knowledge and mutual intelligibility), the fundamental objective of CA is to explore the 'competences that ordinary speakers use and rely on in participating in intelligible, socially organized interaction' (Heritage & Atkinson, 1984, p. 1). Schegloff and Sacks (1973) also stated that

> Our analysis has sought to explicate the ways in which the materials are produced by members in orderly ways that exhibit their orderliness and have their orderliness appreciated and used, and have that appreciation displayed and treated as the basis for subsequent action.
>
> (p. 290)

Basic assumptions underlying this objective are that, on the one hand, there is a common-sense understanding (or intersubjectivity, Heritage, 2013) of the social world that guides people to make sense of their experiences; and on the other hand, the employment of a CA approach requires naturally occurring conversational data based on which orderliness of talk can be defined. Such a specimen approach (Alasuutari, 1995) allows order to emerge from the data. Insofar as it looks for orderliness in interactions, CA's findings are based on the examination of large-scale interactional data (Drew et al., 2001). This convention is preferred in most CA studies, despite the 'relevance of single occasion as the locus of order' (Schegloff, 1987, p. 102). CA researchers believe that by collecting large numbers of instances, some recurrent patterns can be discovered. Data used in CA analysis comprise mainly audio-/video-recordings (Schegloff, 2003). Recordings are transcribed in considerable linguistic and contextual detail to capture the nuances of talk-in-interaction and permit subsequent analysis as such. As Psathas and Anderson (1990) comment, the Jeffersonian Transcription System (Jefferson, 1984, 2004) used for CA makes the transcripts visible.

The tenet of CA is that conversation is sequentially organized and that the sequence of the flow of conversation is constructed by the turn-taking system (Schegloff, 2001). Therefore, much of what CA discusses is the sequential organization of conversation, including the organization of turn-taking, sequences, lexical items, and overall structures. Conversationalists are primarily interested in examining the orderliness inherent in these details and how these details are accountably developed by participants in situated interactions (Sacks et al., 1974). Key to the system of turn-taking is the notion of adjacency pair (Schegloff

& Sacks, 1973). Schegloff and Sacks argued that the orderliness of such adjacency pair sequences is achieved based on 'the recognisability of first pair part status for some utterances' (p. 296). Stated differently, the first pair part and the second pair part form a membership. Examples of adjacency pairs include question–answer, greeting-greeting–leave-taking, and advice-acceptance/declination, to name but a few.

One of the fundamental assumptions of CA is the understanding of talk as an action (Schegloff, 1991). As Heritage (2013, p. 259) stated, 'conversational interaction is structured by an organization of action which is implemented on a turn-by-turn basis'. Central in CA is the organization of turn-taking (Sacks et al., 1974) – the fundamental level of intersubjective understanding (Peräkylä, 2004). In other words, such turn-by-turn 'architecture of intersubjectivity (Heritage, 2013, p. 254) is dependent on the presumed shared understanding between participants regarding the recipient design (Hutchby, 1995; Sacks & Schegloff, 1979) of the turn. Intersubjective understanding also displays the speaker's orientation toward the ongoing action (e.g., topic initiation and shift) as appropriate in the current 'state of talk' (Heritage & Atkinson, 1984, p. 10). Another level of intersubjective understanding concerns the context, which is particularly noticeable in institutional interaction (Peräkylä, 2004).

While initially developed in the study of ordinary conversation, CA has been extended to different forms of institutional contexts (Antaki, 2011a; Arminen, 2005; Drew & Heritage, 1992; Heritage & Clayman, 2010). This is what Antaki (2011b, p. 6) described as 'institutional applied CA'. Unlike earlier CA studies that regard conversation as an institution and investigate how the conversation is constructed by participants based on social norms, this strand of research uses basic CA knowledge as a resource to examine the operation of institutions in talk (Drew et al., 2001; Heritage, 2005). As Antaki (2011b, p. 8) stated, applying CA to the talk of an institution 'puts institutional activity under the microscope'.

The practice of using CA to study social interactions in medical contexts dates back to the late 1970s and 1980s when a group of scholars showed interest in studying the interactions in the medical encounter (e.g., Atkinson & Heath, 1981; Beckman & Frankel, 1984; Frankel, 1984; West, 1984). Recent years have witnessed a considerable extension of CA applications to examine specific activities such as soliciting patient concerns (Heritage & Robinson, 2006; Robinson & Heritage, 2016), patient problem presentation (Heritage & Clayman, 2010; Robinson & Heritage, 2005), diagnosis and treatment (Heritage & McArthur, 2019; Stivers et al., 2018), and discussion of test results (Gutzmer & Beach, 2015). CA has also been applied to examine the overall structure of medical interaction (Heritage, 2011; Robinson, 2003), different activity phases (Boyd & Heritage, 2006; Robinson, 2006), and a particular sequence within an activity (Land et al., 2018; Maynard et al., 2016). Such extensive application of CA to different medical activities and the overall structure of medical interaction reflects the robustness of CA in interpreting how activities are undertaken in medical institutions and how the accomplishment of these activities is supported by the social and institutional norms that are mutually intelligible to both the health provider and the client.

2.4.4 Frame analysis

The concept of frame or framing was introduced by Bateson (1972) and later developed by Goffman (1986) to refer to the basic elements of experience for organizing and making sense of social events. To Bateson, the notion of *frame* is a psychological concept that explains 'how individuals exchange signals that allow them to agree upon the level of abstraction at which any message is intended' (Tannen, 1993b, p. 18). Bateson's (1972) approach was quickly taken up and further developed by scholars in communication, psychology, and sociology. Goffman's (1986) study is a systematic work on the terms, concepts, and the different ways in which segments (or 'strips' using Goffman's term, 1986: 10) of experience are transformed into laminate frames. According to Goffman, the interpretation of social events reflects the primary frameworks that people adopt to understand such events. By identifying frames, people answer questions such as 'what is it that's going on here?' (Goffman, 1986, p. 8). A frame thus describes the implicit rules that shape the meanings generated within the situational event (Berger, 1986). Berger considered the concept of frame as 'a metaphor for what other sociologists have tried to invoke by words like "background", "setting", "context", or a phrase like "in terms of"' (p. xiii). For example, a person sitting on a chair with a cola and popcorn in his hands might evoke the frame of a movie-watching experience. In this sense, frame is metacommunicative in that it provides the listener with instructions in their interpretation of the messages generated within the frame (Bateson, 1972). Frame not only shapes meaning but also organizes the involvement of individuals in the interaction (Goffman, 1986). For instance, frames like classrooms prescribe different involvement between teachers and students in terms of how deeply and fully they are to be carried out into classroom activities.

Frames can be identified by footing – the 'alignment, or set, or stance, or posture, or projected self' that participants 'take up' to themselves and others in the giving and reception of messages (Goffman, 1981, p. 128). During the course of interaction, participants may change their footing, and hence, they change the frame for the ongoing activity. In the chapter entitled 'Footing', Goffman (1981) demonstrated how participants constantly change their footing (e.g., tones, postures, or giving up the floor in a conversation) and how such changes feature in the nature of the talk. Likewise, in medical discussions, participants may change footing through various cues and markers and align themselves to different roles in conversation. For example, Roberts and Sarangi (2005) demonstrated how the doctor's comment on the mother's young daughter, during a physical examination of the baby, introduces the frame of chat and how this doctor-initiated chat also shifts the current footing to reflect a more egalitarian doctor-patient relationship. Frames can also be identified through contextualization cues – any linguistic feature such as code-switching, lexico-grammatical choices, and sequencing that signals the contextual presuppositions of speech activity (Gumperz, 1982). Here, the notion of speech activity is considered as a type of frame. Therefore, the frame theory lies at the core of interactional sociolinguistics (Tannen, 1993a). Gumperz (1982) argued that it is through these contextualization cues that conversationalists are able to make indirect inferences of what is going on here. For example, verbal hesitations and laughter can function as indicators of temporary shifts from the ongoing frame (Beck & Ragan, 1992).

Frame analysis has been successfully applied to studies in healthcare contexts (Tannen & Wallat, 1993; Ribeiro, 1993; Walsh, 2007). Two widely discussed frames are institutional (or medical) and socio-relational (or interpersonal) frames. In a classical study of frame negotiation in medical interactions, Coupland, Robinson, and Coupland (1994) addressed how doctors and elderly patients collaborate in and negotiate the work of entering a medical frame in the opening phase of medical consultation, focusing on sequences generated by doctor's *how-are-you* type of personal state inquiry (Sacks, 1975). In genetic counseling sessions, Sarangi et al. (2011) discussed how genetic counselors invite their clients into decision-making by strategically interweaving different frames over the course of the counseling session. In psychiatric interviews, Ribeiro (2003) examined the interactional asymmetry indexed in participants' negotiation of institutional and interpersonal frames. According to Ribeiro, while the doctor constantly orients to the institutional frame, the patient proposes the interpersonal frame, which features more balanced interpersonal relations. As such, the patient navigates a transition from the sick role (Parsons, 1951) to the role of a person (Mead & Bower, 2000). One consistent finding throughout these studies is the discrepancy in participants' framing priorities in medical encounters. Inspired by these studies, I will combine frame analysis and CA to examine the sequential features of a range of medical activities that reflect participants' framing priorities in different medical encounters.

2.5 Summary

This chapter has argued that there is insufficient understanding of doctor-older patient interaction in chronic care. Chronic diseases are defined as conditions that require ongoing care. While WM is probably the most widely used approach to treat patients with chronic conditions using methods such as drugs, radiation, and surgery, other medical approaches such as TCM are also actively employed in serving these patients. The communication behaviors of doctors and patients in both TCM and WM will be explored in subsequent chapters using both quantitative and qualitative approaches. Patient satisfaction will be reported.

References

Adelman, R. D., Greene, M. G., & Charon, R. (1991). Issues in physician-elderly patient interaction. *Aging and Society, 11*(2), 127–148. https://doi.org/10.1017/S0144686X00003974

Adelman, R. D., Greene, M. G., & Ory, M. G. (2000). Communication between older patients and their physicians. *Clinics in Geriatric Medicine, 16*(1), 1–24. https://doi.org/10.1016/S0749-0690(05)70004-5

Adelman, R. D., Greene, M. G., Charon, R., & Friedman, E. (1992). The content of physician and elderly patient interaction in the medical primary care encounter. *Communication Research, 19*(3), 370–380. https://doi.org/10.1177%2F009365092019003004

Alasuutari, P. (1995). *Researching culture: Qualitative method and cultural studies.* London: SAGE.

Antaki, C. (Ed.). (2011a). *Applied conversation analysis: Intervention and change in institutional talk.* New York: Palgrave Macmillan. https://doi.org/10.1057/9780230316874

Antaki, C. (2011b). Six kinds of applied conversation analysis. In C. Antaki (Ed.), *Applied conversation analysis: Intervention and change in institutional talk* (pp. 1–14). New York: Palgrave Macmillan. https://doi.org/10.1057/9780230316874_1

Arminen, I. (2005). *Institutional interaction: Studies of talk at work.* Surrey: Ashgate. http://dx.doi.org/10.4324/9781315252209

Arora, N. K., & McHorney, C. A. (2000). Patient preferences for medical decision making: Who really wants to participate? *Medical Care, 38*(3), 35–341. https://doi.org/10.1097/00005650-200003000-00010

Atkinson, P., & Heath, C. C. (1981). *Medical work: Realities and routines.* Farnborough: Gower.

Baker, S. C., Watson, B. M., Jamieson, B., & Jamieson, R. (2020). How do patients define satisfaction? The role of patient perceptions of their participation and health provider emotional expression. *Health Communication, 36*(14), 1970–1979. https://doi.org/10.1080/10410236.2020.1808409

Bales, R. F. (1950). *Interaction process analysis.* Cambridge: Addison-Wesley

Barnes, R. K. (2019). Conversation analysis of communication in medical care: Description and beyond. *Research on Language and Social Interaction, 52*(3), 300–315. https://doi.org/10.1080/08351813.2019.1631056

Bateson, G. (1972). *Steps to an ecology of mind.* Northvale, NJ: Jason Aronson.

Beck, C. S., & Ragan, S. L. (1992). Negotiating interpersonal and medical talk: Frame shifts in the gynecologic exam. *Journal of Language and Social Psychology, 11*(1-2), 47–61. https://doi.org/10.1177%2F0261927X92111004

Beckman, H. B., & Frankel, R. M. (1984). The effect of physician behavior on the collection of data. *Annals of Internal Medicine, 101*(5), 692–696. https://doi.org/10.7326/0003-4819-101-5-692

Belcher, V. N., Fried, T. R., Agostini, J. V., & Tinetti, M. E. (2005). Views of older adults on patient participation in medication-related decision making. *Journal of General Internal Medicine, 21*, 298–303. https://doi.org/10.1111/j.1525-1497.2006.00329.x

Berger, B. (1986). Foreword. In E. Goffman. *Frame analysis: An essay on the organization of experience.* Boston: Northeastern University Press.

Boyd, E., & Heritage, J. (2006). Taking the history: Questioning during comprehensive history-taking. In J. Heritage & D. W. Maynard (Eds.), *Communication in medical care: Interaction between primary care physicians and patients* (pp. 151–184). Cambridge University Press. https://doi.org/10.1017/CBO9780511607172.008

Brickley, B., Williams, L. T., Morgan, M., Ross, A., Trigger, K., & Ball, L. (2021). Putting patients first: Development of a patient advocate and general practitioner-informed model of patient-centred care. *BMC Health Services Research, 21*, 261. https://doi.org/10.1186/s12913-021-06273-y

Brown, J. B., Stewart, M., & McWilliam, C. L. (1999). Using the patient-centered method to achieve excellence in care for women with breast cancer. *Patient Education and Counseling, 38*(2), 121–129. https://doi.org/10.1016/S0738-3991(99)00059-2

Burgoon, J. K., & Hale, J. L. (1984). The fundamental topoi of relational communication. *Communication Monographs, 51*(3), 193–214. https://doi.org/10.1080/03637758409390195

Burgoon, J. K., & Hale, J. L. (1987). Validation and measurement of the fundamental themes of relational communication. *Communication Monographs, 54*(1), 19–41. https://doi.org/10.1080/03637758709390214

Burgoon, J. K., Pfau, M., Parrott, R., Birk, T., Coker, R., & Burgoon, M. (1987). Relational communication, satisfaction, compliance-gaining strategies, and compliance in communication between physicians and patients. *Communication Monographs, 54*(3), 307–324. https://doi.org/10.1080/03637758709390235

Burnham, J. C. (2014). Why sociologists abandoned the sick role concept? *History of the Human Sciences, 27*(1), 70–87. https://doi.org/10.1177%2F0952695113507572

Carrard, V., Mast, M. S., Jaunin-Stalder, N., Perron, N. J., & Sommer, J. (2018). Patient-centeredness as physician behavioral adaptability to patient preferences. *Health Communication, 33*(5), 593–600. https://doi.org/10.1080/10410236.2017.1286282

Charon, R., Greene, M. G., & Adelman, R. D. (1994). Multi-dimensional interaction analysis: A collaborative approach to the study of medical discourse. *Social Science & Medicine, 39*(7), 955–965. https://doi.org/10.1016/0277-9536(94)90207-0

Chi, W. C., Wolff, J., Greer, R., & Dy, S. (2017). Multimorbidity and decision-making preferences among older adults. *The Annals of Family Medicine, 15*(6), 546–551. https://doi.org/10.1370/afm.2106

Chiu, C., Feuz, M. A., McMahan, R. D., Miao, Y., & Sudore, R. L. (2016). 'Doctor, make My decisions': Decision control preferences, advance care planning, and satisfaction with communication among diverse older adults. *Journal of Pain and Symptom Management, 51*(1), 33–40. https://doi.org/10.1016/j.jpainsymman.2015.07.018

Chung, C. H., Lau, C. H., Wong, M. C., Yeoh, E. K., & Griffiths, S. M. (2009). Perceived quality of communication amongst outpatients in western and traditional Chinese medicine clinics in a Chinese population. *Health Policy, 90*(1), 66–72. https://doi.org/10.1016/j.healthpol.2008.09.005

Cole, S. A., & Bird, J. (2013). *The medical interview: The three function approach.* Philadelphia: Saunders.

Coupland, J., Robinson, J. D., & Coupland, N. (1994). Frame negotiation in doctor-elderly patient consultations. *Discourse & Society, 5*(1), 89–124. https://doi.org/10.1177%2F0957926594005001005

Daher, M. (2012). Cultural beliefs and values in cancer patients. *Annals of Oncology, 23*(3), iii66–iii99. https://doi.org/10.1093/annonc/mds091

Drew, P., & Heritage, P. (Eds.). (1992). *Talk at work: Interaction in institutional settings.* Cambridge: Cambridge University Press.

Drew, P., Chatwin, J., & Collins, S. (2001). Conversation analysis: A method for research into interactions between patients and health-care professionals. *Health Expectations, 4*(1), 58–70. https://doi.org/10.1046/j.1369-6513.2001.00125.x

Ellington, L., Carlisle, M., & Reblin, M. (2014). Medical interaction analysis systems: Coding challenges when applied to communication in palliative care. In H. E. Hamilton & W-y. S. Chou (Eds.), *The Routledge handbook of language and health communication* (pp. 629–641). London and New York: Routledge.

Fang, Y.-X. (2017). Burnout and work-family conflict among nurses during the preparation for reevaluation of a grade A tertiary hospital. *Chinese Nursing Research, 4*(1), 51–55. https://doi.org/10.1016/j.cnre.2017.03.010

Finkelstein, A., Carmel, S., & Bachner, Y. G. (2017). Physicians' communication styles as correlates of elderly cancer patients' satisfaction with their doctors. *European Journal of Cancer Care, 26*(1), e12399. https://doi.org/10.1111/ecc.12399

Frankel, R. M. (1984). From sentence to sequence: Understanding the medical encounter through microinteractional analysis. *Discourse Processes, 7*(2), 135–170. https://doi.org/10.1080/01638538409544587

Gallagher, T. J., Hartung, P. J., & Gregory Jr., S. W. (2001). Assessment of a measure of relational communication for doctor-patient interactions. *Patient Education and Counseling, 45*(3), 211–218. https://doi.org/10.1016/S0738-3991(01)00126-4

Gan, Y-q., Zheng, L., Yu, N. X., Zhou, G-y., Miao, M., & Lu, Q. (2017). Why do oncologists hide the truth? Disclosure of cancer diagnoses to patients in China: A multisource assessment using mixed methods. *Psycho-Oncology, 27*(5), 1457–1463. https://doi.org/10.1002/pon.4545

Garfinkel, H. (1967) *Studies in ethnomethodology*. Englewood Cliffs, NJ: Prentice-Hall.

Goffman, E. (1981). *Forms of talk*. Philadelphia: University of Pennsylvania Press.

Goffman, E. (1983). The interaction order. *American Sociological Review, 48*(1), 1–17. https://doi.org/10.2307/2095141

Goffman, E. (1986). *Frame analysis: An essay on the organization of experience*. Boston: Northeastern University Press.

Goldfarb, M., & Casillas, J. (2014). Unmet information and support needs in newly diagnosed thyroid cancer: Comparison of adolescents/young adults (AYA) and older patients. *Journal of Cancer Survivorship, 8*, 394–401. https://doi.org/10.1007/s11764-014-0345-7

Greene, M. G., & Adelman, R. (1996). Psychosocial factors in older patients' medical encounters. *Research on Aging, 18*(1), 84–102. https://doi.org/10.1177%2F0164027596181006

Greene, M. G., Adelman, R. D., Charon, R., & Friedmann, E. (1989). Concordance between physicians and their older and younger patients in the primary care medical encounter. *The Gerontologist, 29*(6), 808–813. https://doi.org/10.1093/geront/29.6.808

Greene, M. G., Adelman, R. D., Friedmann, E., & Charon, R. (1994). Older patient satisfaction with communication during an initial medical encounter. *Social Science & Medicine, 38*(9), 1279–1288. https://doi.org/10.1016/0277-9536(94)90191-0

Gu, Y. G. (1996). Doctor-patient interaction as goal-directed discourse in Chinese sociocultural context. *Journal of Asian Pacific Communication, 7*, 156–176.

Gumperz, J. J. (1982). *Discourse strategies*. Cambridge: Cambridge University Press.

Gutzmer, K., & Beach, W. A. (2015). 'Having an ovary this big is not normal': Physicians' use of normal to assess wellness and sickness during oncology interviews. *Health Communication, 30*(1), 8–18. https://doi.org/10.1080/10410236.2014.881176

Hall, J. A., Roter, D. L., & Katz, N. R. (1987). Task versus socio-emotional behaviors in physicians. *Medical Care, 25*(5), 399–412. https://doi.org/10.1097/00005650-198705000-00004

Haug, M. R., & Ory, M. G. (1987). Issues in elderly patient-provider interactions. *Research on Aging, 9*(1), 3–44. https://doi.org/10.1177%2F0164027587009001001

Heritage, J. (2005). Conversation analysis and institutional talk. In K. L. Fitch & R. E. Sanders (Eds.), *Handbook of language and social interaction* (pp. 233–331). Mahwah, NJ: Lawrence Erlbaum Associates.

Heritage, J. (2011). The interaction order and clinical practice: Some observations on dysfunctions and action steps. *Patient Education and Counseling, 84*(3), 338–343. https://doi.org/10.1016/j.pec.2011.05.022

Heritage, J. (2013). *Garfinkel and ethnomethodology.* Cambridge: Polity Press.

Heritage, J., & Atkinson, J. M. (1984). Introduction. In J. M. Atkinson & J. Heritage (Eds.), *Structures of social action: Studies in conversation analysis* (pp. 1–15). Cambridge: Cambridge University Press.

Heritage, J., & Clayman, S. (2010). *Talk in action: Interactions, identities, and institutions.* Oxford: Wiley-Blackwell.

Heritage, J., & Maynard, D. W. (2006). Introduction: Analyzing interaction between doctors and patients in primary care encounters. In J. Heritage & D. W. Maynard (Eds.), *Communication in medical care: Interaction between primary care physicians and patients* (pp.1–21). Cambridge: Cambridge University Press. https://doi.org/10.1017/CBO9780511607172.003

Heritage, J., & McArthur, A. (2019). The diagnostic moment: A study in US primary care. *Social Science & Medicine, 228,* 262–271. https://doi.org/10.1016/j.socscimed.2019.03.022

Heritage, J., & Robinson, J. D. (2006). The structure of patients' presenting concerns: Physicians' opening questions. *Health Communication, 19*(2), 89–102. https://doi.org/10.1207/s15327027hc1902_1

Hobbs, J. L. (2009). A dimensional analysis of patient-centered care. *Nursing Research, 58*(1), 52–62. https://doi.org/10.1097/NNR.0b013e31818c3e79

Hoffmann, T., Jansen, J., & Glasziou, P. (2018). The importance and challenges for shared decision making in older people with multimorbidity. *PLoS Medicine, 15*(3), e1002530. https://doi.org/10.1371/journal.pmed.1002530

Hougaard, J. L., Østerdal, L. P., & Yu, Y. (2011). The Chinese healthcare system: Structure, problems and challenges. *Applied Health Economics and Health Policy, 9,* 1–13. https://doi.org/10.2165/11531800-000000000-00000

Hu, Y-h., & Zhang, Z-x. (2015). Skilled doctors in tertiary hospitals are already overworked in China. *The Lancet Global Health, 3*(12), e737. https://doi.org/10.1016/S2214-109X(15)00192-8

Hudon, C., Fortin, M., Haggerty, J., Loignon, C., Lambert, M., & Poitras, M-E. (2012). Patient-centered care in chronic disease management: A thematic analysis of the literature in family medicine. *Patient Education and Counseling, 88*(2), 170–176. https://doi.org/10.1016/j.pec.2012.01.009

Hutchby, I. (1995). Aspects of recipient design in expert advice-giving on call-in radio. *Discourse Processes, 19*(2), 219–238. http://dx.doi.org/10.1080/01638539509544915

Inui, T. S., Carter, W. B., Kukull, W. A., & Haign, V. H. (1982). Outcome-based doctor-patient interaction analysis I: Comparison of techniques. *Medical Care, 20*(6), 535–549. https://doi.org/10.1097/00005650-198206000-00001

Jefferson, G. (1984). Transcription notation. In J. M. Atkinson & J. Heritage (Eds.), *Structures of social action* (pp. ix–xvi). Cambridge and New York: Cambridge University Press.

Jefferson, G. (2004). Glossary of transcript symbols with an introduction. In G. H. Lerner (Eds.), *Conversation analysis: Studies from the first generation* (pp. 13–31). Philadelphia: John Benjamins. https://doi.org/10.1075/pbns.125.02jef

Koenig, C. J., & Robinson, J. D. (2014). Conversation analysis: Understanding the structure of health talk. In B. B. Whaley (Ed.), *Research methods in health communication: Principles and application* (pp. 119–140). New York: Routledge.

Korsch, B. M., & Negrete, V. F. (1972). Doctor-patient communication. *Scientific American, 227*, 66–74. https://doi.org/10.1038/scientificamerican0872-66

Korsch, B. M., Gozzi, E. K., & Francis, V. (1968). Gaps in doctor-patient communication. *Pediatrics, 42*(5), 855–871.

Kuluski, K., Gill, A., Naganathan, G., Upshur, R., Jaakkimainen, R. L., & Wodchis, W. P. (2013). A qualitative descriptive study on the alignment of care goals between older persons with multimorbidities, their family physicians and informal care givers. *BMC Family Practice, 14*, 133. https://doi.org/10.1186/1471-2296-14-133

Kuluski, K., Peckham, A., Gill, A., Gagnon, D., Wong-Cornall, C., McKillop, A., Parsons, J., & Sheridan, N. (2019). What is important to older people with multimorbidity and their caregivers? Identifying attributes of person centered care from the user perspective. *International Journal of Integrated Care, 19*(3), 4. http://doi.org/10.5334/ijic.4655

Land, V., Parry, R., Pino, M., Jenkins, L., Feathers, L., & Faull, C. (2018). Addressing possible problems with patients' expectations, plans and decisions for the future: One strategy used by experienced clinicians in advance care planning conversations. *Patient Education and Counselling, 102*(4), 670–679. https://doi.org/10.1016/j.pec.2018.11.008

Levinson, W., Kao, A., Kuby, A., & Thisted, R. A. (2005). Not all patients want to participate in decision making. *Journal of General Internal Medicine, 20*(6), 531–535. https://doi.org/10.1111/j.1525-1497.2005.04101.x

Liang, W-c., Kasman, D., Wang, J. H., Yuan, E. H., & Mandelblatt, J. S. (2006). Communication between older women and physicians: Preliminary implications for satisfaction and intention to have mammography. *Patient Education and Counseling, 64*(1–3), 387–392. https://doi.org/10.1016/j.pec.2006.04.004

Little, P., Everitt, H., Williamson, I., Warner, G., Moore, M., Gould, C., Ferrier, K., & Payne, S. (2001). Preferences of patients for patient centered approach to consultation in primary care: Observational study. *BMJ, 322*, 468–472. https://doi.org/10.1136/bmj.322.7284.468

Liu, Y-x., Yang, J-h., Huo, D., Fan, H-h., Gao, Y-f. (2018). Disclosure of cancer diagnosis in China: The incidence, patients' situation, and different preferences between patients and their family members and related influence factors. *Cancer Management and Research, 10*, 2173–2181. https://doi.org/10.2147/CMAR.S166437

Maly, R. C., Leake, B., Frank, J. C., DiMatteo, M. R., & Reuben, D. B. (2002). Implementation of consultative geriatric recommendations: The role of patient-primary care physician concordance. *Journal of the American Geriatrics Society, 50*(8), 1372–1380. https://doi.org/10.1046/j.1532-5415.2002.50358.x

Marcinowicz, L., Pawlikowska, T., & Oleszczyk, M. (2014). What do older people value when they visit their general practitioner? A qualitative study. *European Journal of Aging, 11*, 361–367. https://doi.org/10.1007/s10433-014-0313-0

Maynard, D. W., Cortez, D., & Campbell, T. C. (2016). End of life conversations, appreciation sequences, and the interaction order in cancer clinics. *Patient Education and Counseling, 99*(1), 92–100. https://doi.org/10.1016/j.pec.2015.07.015

Mead, N., & Bower, P. (2000). Patient-centeredness: A conceptual framework and review of the empirical literature. *Social Science & Medicine, 51*(7), 1087–1110. https://doi.org/10.1016/S0277-9536(00)00098-8

Mishler, E. G. (1984). *The discourse of medicine: Dialectics of medical interviews*. Norwood, NJ: Ablex.

Mitina, M., Young, S., Zhavoronkov, A. (2020). Psychological aging, depression, and well-being. *Aging, 12*(18), 18765–18777. https://doi.org/10.18632/aging.103880

Naik, A. D., Martin, L. A., Moye, J., & Karel, M. J. (2016). Health values and treatment goals of older multimorbid adults facing life-threatening illness. *Journal of the American Geriatrics Society, 64*(3), 625–631. https://doi.org/10.1111/jgs.14027

Ong, L. M. L., De Haes, J. C. J. M., Hoos, A. M., & Lammes, F. B. (1995). Doctor-patient communication: A review of the literature. *Social Science & Medicine, 40*(7), 903–918. https://doi.org/10.1016/0277-9536(94)00155-M

Ong, L. M. L., Visser, M. R. M., Kruyver, I. P. M., Bensing, J. M., Brink-Muinen, A. V. D., Stouthhard, J. M. L., Lammes, F. B., & de Haes, J. C. J. M. (1998). The Roter Interaction Analysis System (RIAS) in oncological consultations: Psychometric properties. *Psycho-Oncology, 7*(5), 387–401. https://doi.org/10.1002/(SICI)1099-1611(1998090)7:5%3C387::AID-PON316%3E3.0.CO;2-G

Parsons, T. (1951). *The social system.* London: Routledge.

Parsons, T. (1975). The sick role and the role of the physician reconsidered. *The Milbank Memorial Fund Quarterly. Health and Society, 53*(3), 257–278. https://doi.org/10.2307/3349493

Pelicano-Romano, J., Neves, M. R., Amado, A., & Cavaco, A. M. (2013). Do community pharmacists actively engage elderly patients in the dialogue? Results from pharmaceutical care consultations. *Health Expectations, 18*(5), 1721–1734. https://doi.org/10.1111/hex.12165

Pel-Little, R. E., Snaterse, M., Teppich, N. M., Buurman, B. M., van Etten-Jamaludin, F. S., van Weert, J. C. M., Minkman, M. M., & Scholte op Reimer, W. J. M. (2021). Barriers and facilitators for shared decision making in older patients with multiple chronic conditions: A systematic review. *BMC Geriatrics, 21*, 112. https://doi.org/10.1186/s12877-021-02050-y

Peräkylä, A. (2004). Two traditions of interaction research. *British Journal of Social Psychology, 43*(1), 1–20. https://doi.org/10.1348/014466604322915953

Phillips, K. L., Chiriboga, D. A., & Jang, Y. (2012). Satisfaction with care: The role of patient-provider racial/ethnic concordance and interpersonal sensitivity. *Journal of Aging and Health, 24*(7), 1079–1090. https://doi.org/10.1177%2F0898264312453068

Plewnia, A., Bengel, J., & Körner, M. (2016). Patient-centeredness and its impact on patient satisfaction and treatment outcomes in medical rehabilitation. *Patient Education and Counseling, 99*(12), 2063–2070. https://doi.org/10.1016/j.pec.2016.07.018

Psathas, G., & Anderson, T. (1990). The 'practices' of transcription in conversation analysis. *Semiotica, 78*(1/2), 75–99. https://doi.org/10.1515/semi.1990.78.1-2.75

Radley, A. (2004). *Making sense of illness: The social psychology of health and disease.* London: Sage. http://dx.doi.org/10.4135/9781446222287

Ribeiro, B. T. (1993). Framing in psychotic discourse. In D. Tannen (Ed.), *Framing in discourse* (pp. 77–113). Oxford: Oxford University Press.

Ribeiro, B. T. (2003). Conflict talk in psychiatric discharge interview: Struggling between personal and official footings. In C. R. Caldas-Coulthard & M. Coulthard (Eds.), *Texts and practices: Readings in critical discourse analysis* (pp. 179–193). New York: Routledge.

Roberts, C., & Sarangi, S. (2005). Theme-oriented discourse analysis of medical encounters. *Medical Education, 39*(6), 632–640. https://doi.org/10.1111/j.1365-2929.2005.02171.x

Robinson, J. D. (2003). An interactional structure of medical activities during acute visits and its implications for patients' participation. *Health Communication, 15*(1), 27–57. https://doi.org/10.1207/S15327027HC1501_2

Robinson, J. D. (2006). Soliciting patients' presenting concerns. In J. Heritage & D. W. Maynard (Eds.), *Communication in medical care: Interaction between primary care physicians and patients* (pp. 22–47). Cambridge: Cambridge University Press. https://doi.org/10.1017/CBO9780511607172.004

Robinson, J. D., & Heritage, J. (2005). The structure of patients' presenting concerns: The completion relevance of current symptoms. *Social Science & Medicine, 61*(2), 481–493. https://doi.org/10.1016/j.socscimed.2004.12.004

Robinson, J. D., & Heritage, J. (2016). How patients understand physicians' solicitations of additional concerns: implications for up-front agenda setting in primary care. *Health Communication, 31*(4), 434–444. https://doi.org/10.1080/10410236. 2014.960060

Roter, D. L. (1977). *The Roter method of interaction process analysis (RIAS manual).* Baltimore: Johns Hopkins University Press.

Roter, D. L. (2010). The Roter Interaction Analysis System (RIAS): Applicability within the context of cancer and palliative care. In D. W. Kissane, B. D. Bultz, P. N. Butow, & I. G. Finlay (Eds.), *Handbook of communication in oncology and palliative care* (pp. 717–726). New York: Oxford University Press. https://doi.org/10.1093/acprof:oso/ 9780199238361.003.0062

Roter, D. L., & Hall, J. A. (1991). Health education theory: An application to the process of patient-provider communication. *Health Education Research, 6*(2), 185–193. https://psycnet.apa.org/doi/10.1093/her/6.2.185

Roter, D. L., & Larson, S. (2001). The relationship between residents' and attending physicians' communication during primary care visits: An illustrative use of the Roter Interaction Analysis System. *Health Communication, 13*(1), 33–48. https://doi.org/ 10.1207/S15327027HC1301_04

Roter, D. L., & Larson, S. (2002). The Roter Interaction Analysis System (RIAS): Utility and flexibility for analysis of medical interactions. *Patient Education and Counseling, 46*(4), 243–251. https://doi.org/10.1016/S0738-3991(02)00012-5

Roter, D. L., Geller, G., Bernhardt, B. A., Larson, S. M., & Doksum, T. (1999). Effects of obstetrician gender on communication and patient satisfaction. *Obstetrics & Gynecology, 93*, 635–641. https://doi.org/10.1016/s0029-7844(98)00542-0

Roter, D. L., Hall, J. A., & Katz, N. R. (1987). Relations between physicians' behaviors and analogue patients' satisfaction, recall, and impressions. *Medical Care, 25*(5), 437– 451. https://psycnet.apa.org/doi/10.1097/00005650-198705000-00007

Sacks, H. (1975). Everyone has to lie. In M. Sanches & B. G. Blount (Eds.), *Sociocultural dimensions of language use* (pp. 57–80). New York: Academic.

Sacks, H., & Schegloff, E. A. (1979). Two preferences in the organization of reference to persons in conversation and their interaction. In G. Psathas (Ed.), *Everyday language: Studies in ethnomethodology* (pp. 15–21). New York: Irvington Publishers. http://dx.doi.org/10.1017/CBO9780511486746.003

Sacks, H., Schegloff, E. A., & Jefferson, G. (1974). A simplest systematics for the organization of turn-taking for conversation. *Language, 50*(4), 696–735. https://doi.org/ 10.2307/412243

Saha, S., & Beach, M. C. (2011). The impact of patient-centered communication on patients' decision making and evaluations of physicians: A randomized study using video vignettes. *Patient Education and Counseling, 84*(3), 386–392. https://doi.org/ 10.1016/j.pec.2011.04.023

Sandvik, M., Eide, H., Lind, M., Graugaard, P. K., Torper, J., & Finset, A. (2002). Analyzing medical dialogues: Strength and weakness of Roter's Interaction Analysis System (RIAS). *Patient Education and Counseling, 46*(4), 235–241. https://doi.org/ 10.1016/S0738-3991(02)00014-9

Sarangi, S., Brookes-Howell, L., Bennert, K., & Clarke, A. (2011). Psychological and sociomoral frames in genetic counseling for predictive testing. In C. N. Candlin & S. Sarangi (Eds.), *Handbook of communication in organizations and professions* (pp. 235–257). Berlin: De Gruyter Mouton. https://doi.org/10.1515/9783110214222.235

Schegloff, E. A. (1987). Analyzing single episodes of interaction: An exercise in conversation analysis. *Social Psychology Quarterly, 50*(2), 101–114. https://psycnet.apa.org/doi/10.2307/2786745

Schegloff, E. A. (1991). Reflections on talk and social structure. In D. Boden & D. H. Zimmerman (Eds.), *Talk and social structure: Studies in ethnomethodology and conversation analysis* (pp. 44–70). Oakland: University of California Press.

Schegloff, E. A. (2001). Discourse as an interactional achievement III: The omnirelevance of action. *Research on Language and Social Interaction, 28*(3), 185–211. https://doi.org/10.1207/s15327973rlsi2803_2

Schegloff, E. A. (2003). On conversation analysis: An interview with Emanuel A. Schegloff with Světla Cmejrkov and Carlo, L. Prevignano. In C. L. Prevignano & Thibault, P. J. (Eds.), *Discussing conversation analysis: The work of Emanuel A. Schegloff* (pp. 11–55). Amsterdam: John Benjamins. https://doi.org/10.1075/z.118.03cme

Schegloff, E. A., & Sacks, H. (1973). Opening up closings. *Semiotica, 8*, 289–327. https://doi.org/10.1515/semi.1973.8.4.289

Schulman-Green, D. J., Naik, A. D., Bradley, E. H., McCorkle, R., & Bogardus, S. T. (2006). Goal setting as a shared decision making strategy among clinicians and their older patients. *Patient Education and Counseling, 63*(1–2), 145–151. https://doi.org/10.1016/j.pec.2005.09.010

Schumacher, S., Rief, W., Brähler, E., Martin, A., Glaesmer, H., & Mewes, R. (2013). Disagreement in doctor's and patient's rating about medically unexplained symptoms and health care use. *International Journal of Behavioral Medicine, 20*, 30–37. https://doi.org/10.1007/s12529-011-9213-2

Stewart, M. (2001): Towards a global definition of patient centered care: The patient should be the judge of patient centered care. *BMJ, 322*, 444–445. https://doi.org/10.1136/bmj.322.7284.444

Stewart, M., Brown, J. B., Weson, W. W., McWhinney, I. R., McWilliam, C. L., & Freeman, T. R. (2003). *Patient-centered medicine: Transforming the clinical method.* Abingdon: Redcliffe Medical Press.

Stewart, M., Meredith, L., Brown, J. B., & Galajda, J. (2000). The influence of older patient-physician communication on health and health-related outcomes. *Clinics in Geriatric Medicine, 16*(1), 25–36. https://doi.org/10.1016/S0749-0690(05)70005-7

Stiles, W. B. (1981). Classification of intersubjective illocutionary acts. *Language in Society, 10*(2), 227–249.

Stivers, T., Heritage, J., Barnes, R. K., McCabe, R., Thompson, L., & Toerien, M. (2018). Treatment recommendations as actions. *Health Communication, 33*(11), 1335–1344. https://doi.org/10.1080/10410236.2017.1350913

Tannen, D. (1993a). Introduction. In D. Tannen (Ed.), *Framing in discourse* (pp. 3–13). Oxford: Oxford University Press.

Tannen, D. (1993b). What's in a frame? Surface evidence for underlying expectations. In D. Tannen (Ed.), *Framing in discourse* (pp. 14–56). Oxford: Oxford University Press.

Tannen, D., & Wallat, C. (1993). Interactive frames and knowledge schemas in interaction: Examples from a medical examination/interview. In D. Tannen (Ed.), *Framing in discourse* (pp. 57–76). Oxford: Oxford University Press.

Tse, C. Y., Chong, A., & Fok, S. Y. (2013). Breaking bad news: A Chinese perspective. *Palliative Medicine, 17*(4), 339–343. https://doi.org/10.1191%2F026921 6303pm751oa

van Weert, J. C. M., Bolle, S., van Dulmen, S., & Jansen, J. (2013). Older cancer patients' information and communication needs: What they want is what they get? *Patient Education and Counseling, 92*(3), 388–397. https://doi.org/10.1016/j.pec. 2013.03.011

Varul, M. Z. (2010). Talcott Parsons, the sick role and chronic illness. *Body & Society, 16*(2), 72–94. https://doi.org/10.1177%2F1357034X10364766

Vermunt, N. P., Harmsen, M., Elwyn, G., Westert, G. P., Burgers, J. S., Olde Rikkert, M. G., & Faber, M. J. (2017). A three-goal model for patients with multimorbidity: A qualitative approach. *Health Expectations, 21*(2), 528–538. https://doi.org/10.1111/hex.12647

Walsh, I. P. (2007). Small talk is 'big talk' in clinical discourse: Appreciating the value of conversation in SLP clinical interactions. *Topics in Language Disorders, 27*(1), 24–36. http://dx.doi.org/10.1097/00011363-200701000-00004

Wang, Q. (2010). *Doctor–patient communication and patient satisfaction: A crosscultural comparative study between China and the US* (Publication No. 3444876) [Doctoral Dissertation, Purdue University]. ProQuest Dissertations and Theses Database.

Ware Jr., J. E., Davies-Avery, A., & Stewart, A. L. (1978). The measurement and meaning of patient satisfaction: A review of the literature. *Health and Medical Care Services Review, 1*(1), 1–15.

West, C. (1984). *Routine complications: Troubles with talk between doctors and patients.* Bloomington: Indiana University Press.

Wissow, L. S., Roter, D., Bauman, L. J., Crain, E., Kercsmar, C., Weiss, K., Mitchell, H., & Mohr, B. (1998). Patient-provider communication during the emergency department care of children with asthma. *Medical Care, 36*(10), 1439–1450. https://doi. org/10.1097/00005650-199810000-00002

Wu, V. S., Smith, A. B., & Girgis, A. (2020). The unmet supportive care needs of Chinese patients and caregivers affected by cancer: A systematic review [Special issue]. *European Journal of Cancer Care,* Special Issue article, e13269. https://doi.org/10.1111/ecc.13269

Yi, T-w., Deng, Y-t., Chen, H-p., Zhang, J., Liu, J., Huang, B-y., Wang, Y-q., Jiang, Y. (2016). The discordance of information needs between cancer patients and their families in China. *Patient Education and Counseling, 99*(5), 863–869. https://doi.org/10.1016/j.pec.2015.12.022

3   Interaction analysis

3.1 Introduction

A widely used dichotomy in understanding doctor–patient communication is the distinction between instrumental and affective behaviors. Studies have suggested that these two broad categories of communication meet patients' information needs for cure and interpersonal needs for care (Ong et al., 1995). In my review of the literature, I noted that while numerous attempts have been made by scholars in observing participants' performance in these two domains of communication, most of the earlier studies focus on primary care encounters. There are also relatively few studies comparing participants' communication in different types of care providers.

This chapter is a quantitative study of participants' verbal behaviors in TCM and WM encounters. The study mainly uses RIAS codes to categorize and quantify doctor and patient interactions at different levels (e.g., instrumental and socio-emotional). The unit of analysis is the utterance, defined as 'the smallest discriminable speech segment […] which expresses or implies a complete thought' (Roter et al. 1987, p. 440). In that sense, an utterance can be as short as a word or as long as a sentence. In Chapter 2, I briefly discussed the development of RIAS, weighed its strengths and weaknesses in examining medical interactions, and reviewed studies applying RIAS to different medical contexts. In this chapter, I first discuss the coding conventions and methods, illustrated with examples. I turn in the second half of the chapter to the results and findings, where I highlight the similarities and differences between TCM and WM in relation to communication behaviors.

3.2 Coding conventions and calculation of utterances

RIAS (Roter, 1977) was used to code the 69 medial consultations (see Figures 3.1 and 3.2) based on the content and function of the utterance. The challenge is understanding the function of utterances. One feature of talk-in-interaction is that an utterance can be multifunctional. For example, while the articulation of *how-are-you* can be taken as phatic and relational greetings, it can also be understood as a serious medically associated diagnostic elicitation (Coupland et al.,

DOI: 10.4324/9781003161929-3

1992). To solve this dilemma, I consider the immediate sequential position of the utterance and the recipient's response.

The RIAS codes were pretested by 45 older adults for their completeness and clarity. Test-retest reliability (one-month interval) score was 0.9. While most of the codes can capture the content and function of participants' utterances, I distinguish diagnostic tests from medical conditions. In the original RIAS codes (Roter, 1977), statements in relation to medical conditions, diagnosis, previous tests, and test results were all coded as *medical conditions*. Yet, this categorization was less effective in capturing participants' priority in information-seeking and giving in the pilot study. Utterances relating to diagnostic tests and test results in WM visits far outnumbered those in TCM visits. I concur that information about diagnostic tests is crucial to patients' medical conditions. However, the inclusiveness of *medical conditions* greatly limits understanding the disparity between TCM and WM in relation to the type of information. Therefore, the original RIAS codes were modified to include *diagnostic tests* as a content code (see Figures 3.1 and 3.2). To avoid overlaps, utterances with explicit content of diagnostic tests (e.g., tests that were recommended by doctors at the time of consultation or discussions concerning the health indices on the patient's earlier diagnostic test reports) were coded as diagnostic tests rather than medical conditions. The criteria to code an utterance as diagnostic tests is the explicitness of the test or the health indices.

Questions in this study were defined based on adjacency pair principles (Schegloff & Sacks, 1973), that is, expecting an answer. In that sense, an utterance like '你怎麼不好' (*What's wrong?*) was coded as open questions, and one like '睡眠還可以吧' (*Do you sleep well?*) was coded as closed-ended questions. The content of the question was coded into two broad categories of biomedical and lifestyle/psychosocial. Biomedical topics include discussions on medical conditions (e.g., '有藥物過敏嗎' *any drug allergies?*), diagnostic tests (e.g., '胃鏡在哪裡做的' *Where did you have the gastroscopy?*), and therapeutic regimens (e.g., '做不做手術' *Do you want the surgery or not?*). While such questions initiated by the doctor were clustered into the category of data collection, questions of this nature initiated by the patient were conceptualized as information-seeking (see Roter, 1984). Patient-initiated questions articulated for a particular service such as medication refills (e.g., '醫生有沒有中藥幫我配一點' *Doctor, may I take some herbal medicine?*) were coded as requesting service. Questions articulated for checking understanding were excluded from this category and were treated as facilitation statements (to be discussed). Answers to questions were coded as information-giving, mostly instantiated via declarative statements.

While questions and information-giving are codes that describe the behaviors of both the doctor and the patient, patient counseling is a code reserved for the doctor. Patient counseling is similar to information-giving in that both include statements that assist patients in making sense of their health conditions and coping with various demands for treatment (Roter & Hall, 2004). The distinction between the two behaviors is that while information-giving is mainly

Data gathering
- Closed questions
  - Biomedical (medical condition; therapeutics; diagnostic tests; others)
  - Lifestyle/psychosocial
- Open questions
  - Lifestyle/psychosocial
  - Biomedical (medical condition; therapeutics; diagnostic tests; others)

Information-giving & counseling
- Giving information
  - Lifestyle/psychosocial
  - Biomedical (medical condition; therapeutics; diagnostic tests; others)
- Counseling
  - Lifestyle/psychosocial
  - Biomedical (therapeutics; diagnostic tests)

Relationship building
- Positive talk
  - Approval
  - Agreement
- Negative talk
  - Criticism
  - Disapproval
- Social conversation
  - Laughs
  - Jokes
  - Chitchat
- Emotional talk
  - Concern / worry
  - Reassurance
  - Legitimacy
  - Empathy
  - Self-disclosure

Partnership building
- Verbal attentiveness
  - Showing understanding
  - Backchannel
- Procedural
  - Transition
  - Giving directions
- Facilitation
  - Checks
  - Bid for repetition
  - Ask for opinion

Missing value
- Unintelligible
- Unfinished

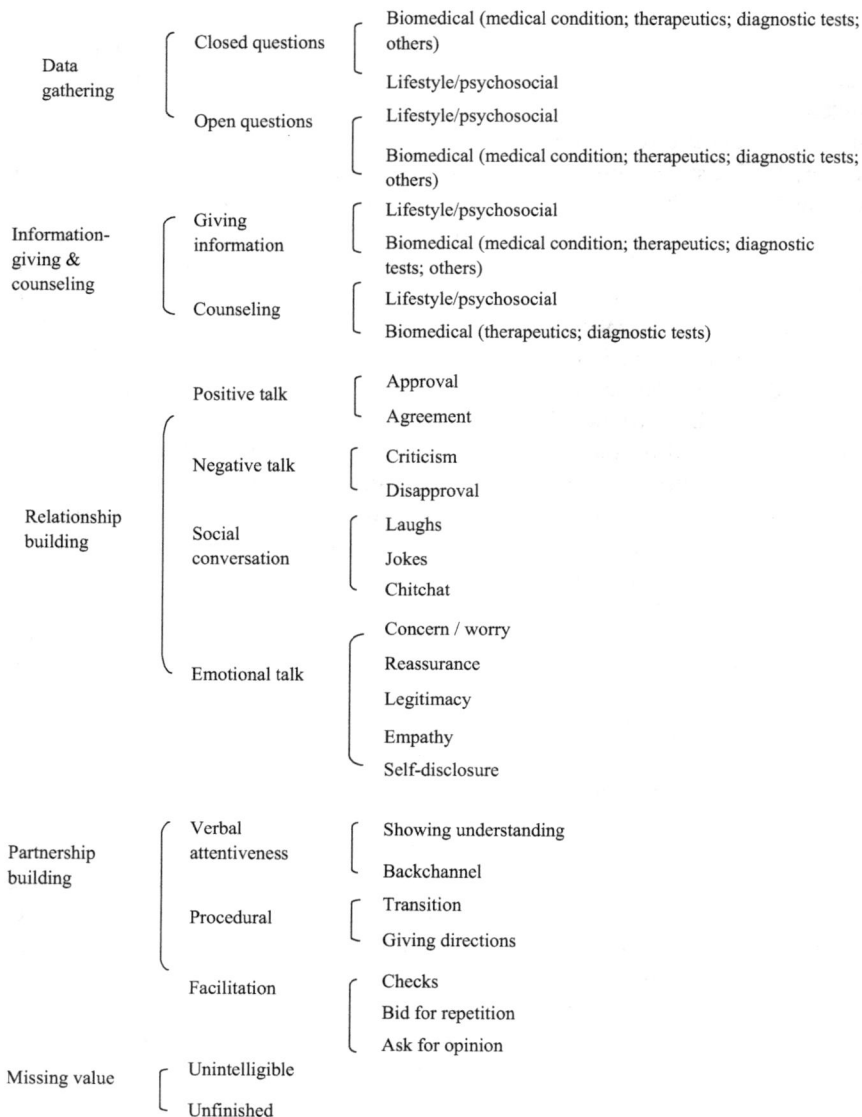

Figure 3.1 RIAS codes for the doctor.

Data gathering
- Closed questions
  - Biomedical (medical condition; therapeutic regimen; diagnostic tests; others)
  - Lifestyle/psychosocial
- Open questions
  - Lifestyle/psychosocial
  - Biomedical (medical condition; therapeutic regimen; diagnostic tests; others)
- Request for service

Information giving
- Biomedical (medical condition; therapeutic regimen; diagnostic tests; others)
- Lifestyle/psychosocial

Relationship building
- Positive talk
  - Approval
  - Agreement
- Negative talk
  - Criticism
  - Disapproval
- Social conversation
  - Laughs
  - Chitchat
- Emotional talk
  - Concern / worry
  - Seeking reassurance
  - Legitimacy
  - Empathy

Partnership building
- Verbal attentiveness —— Paraphrasing
- Procedural
  - Transition
  - Giving directions
- Facilitation
  - Checks
  - Bid for repetition
  - Ask for opinion

Missing value
- Unfinished
- Unintelligible

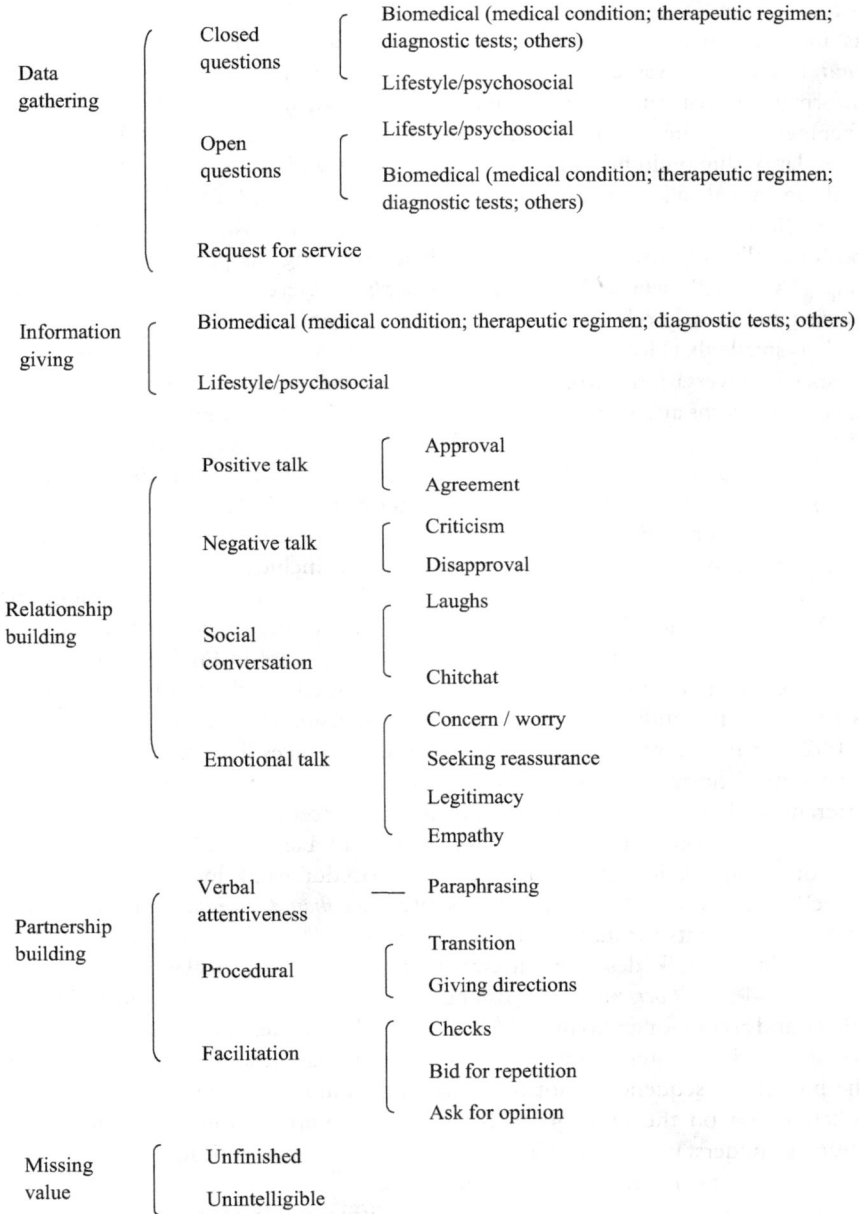

Figure 3.2 RIAS codes for the patient.

explanatory, counseling is more persuasive and advisory in nature. Therefore, an utterance like '你血糖有點高' (*Your blood glucose levels have increased*) was coded as information-giving, whereas a statement like '要控制一下米飯哦' (*Watch your rice intake*) was coded as patient counseling. The topics of participants' information-giving include medical conditions (e.g., symptoms), diagnostic tests, therapeutic regimen, and lifestyle/psychosocial issues (e.g., stress and family).

Relationship building consists of positive and negative talk, social conversation, and emotional talk. Statements showing approval (e.g., '你的努力還是有用的' *Your efforts are rewarded*) and agreement (e.g., '好的' *okay*) are considered as positive talk. Statements of negative valence showing disapproval and criticism (e.g., '早點不說' *why didn't you tell me earlier?*) were coded as negative talk. Statements loosely related to the institutional agenda of the medical interview, such as small talk (Holmes, 2000), laughter and jokes (Ragan, 2000), were coded as social conversation. Utterances that convey the speaker's emotional process, such as concerns and worries (e.g., '那你受不了' *You cannot bear it*), reassurance ('不要緊的' *It matters not*), legitimacy ('這也正常' *It doesn't matter*), empathy ('可憐啊' *Poor you*), and self-disclosure ('我也有的' *I also had a similar experience*) were coded as emotional talk (see Roter & Hall, 2004).

Partnership-building describes talk that encourages the recipient's active engagement in the undergoing interaction. It includes verbal attentiveness such as backchannels (e.g., '嗯' *um*), paraphrasing, and statements indicate understanding (e.g., '我知道了' *Got it*). In Chinese, the articulation of '嗯' can also be interpreted as showing agreement (similar to *yeah* in English), depending on the context. One criterion in discerning a backchannel from the agreement is that the latter indicates a floor shift (see Hayashi, 1991). Roter and Larson (2002) further pointed out that, while some utterances like 'yeah', 'right', and 'mmm-huh' normally function as backchannels, when they occur in patients' utterances, their primary function is to indicate acceptance and agreement. For this consideration, this study follows Roter and Larson's (2002) convention by not coding patient backchannels. The procedural talk includes transitional speech (e.g., '所以你就是說什麼呢' *So what you should do is …*) and directions that guide patients through the consultation (e.g., '嘴巴張開' *open your mouth*). The facilitative talk describes utterances articulated for checking information ('好多了是吧' *It's better, right?*), asking for a repeat of what was said ('什麼啊' *what*), and asking for an opinion ('好嗎' *okay?*). While these facilitative statements are phrased in an interrogative form and hearable as questions, their function in the immediate sequence is not to request new information but rather to invite collaboration on the undergoing project, for example, to invite repair (Chui, 1996) in understanding an object, a phenomenon, or an attitude. In this study, these utterances are separated from questions.

The kappa coefficient was measured for different communication behaviors by Nvivo and further averaged across the five clusters of data gathering, information-giving and counseling (doctor only), information-giving (patient only), relationship-building, and partnership-building. Table 3.1 is a modification of the output for illustration purposes.

Table 3.1 Kappa coefficient for participants' communication clusters

Communication behaviors	Doctor speech	Patient speech
Data gathering	0.92	0.91
Information-giving and counseling	0.92	N/A
Information-giving	N/A	0.93
Relationship building	0.96	0.87
Partnership building	0.92	0.83

Each participant's contribution reflected in RIAS codes was summed up and then calculated into rates. This step is explained by the following formula:

$$R = \frac{x}{y},$$

where R represents the proportion of a participant's contribution in one RIAS category in every single interaction; x represents the number of the participant's utterances in this category; and y represents the total number of that participant's utterances in the current interaction. I use proportion rather than raw frequency to minimize the potential influence caused by the differences in speakers' speaking rate and words per minute and the consultation length.

3.3 Results

3.3.1 Some descriptives of doctor–patient communication

In TCM, the average number of patient utterances was 66 (SD = 37), and the average number of doctor utterances was 49 (SD = 23). In WM, doctors and patients' contribution was relatively similar: the average number of patient utterances was 52 (SD = 32), and the average number of doctor utterances was 53 (SD = 24).

In this study, since the RIAS codes in the doctor's speech were not multivariate normal, a more effective MANOVA model could not be applied to all variables. A closer investigation of the univariate normality shows that while doctors' information-giving and counseling behavior failed to meet the null hypothesis of normal distribution in WM, other behaviors were normally distributed. In the patient's speech, only the information-giving behavior was normally distributed in both TCM and WM visits. Given the observations, non-parametric tests were used where appropriate.

Results of Hotelling's T-square were significant between TCM and WM for both doctor ($T^2 = 106.26$, $F = 25.38$, $df = 4$, 65; $p < 0.01$) and patient speech ($T^2 = 29.95$, $F = 7.16$, $df = 4$, 65; $p < 0.01$), indicating a difference in communication at the level of behavior clusters. Results of univariate F tests are given below in the discussion of specific behaviors. Tables 3.2 and 3.3 report the mean rates (R in the formula) and standard deviations of participants' behaviors.

Table 3.2 Doctor communication results

Behavior clusters	Categories	TCM		WM	
		Mean rates	Std.	Mean rates	Std.
Instrumental	Overall**	0.57	0.11	0.71	0.08
Data collection	Overall**	0.31	0.14	0.16	0.09
	Biomedical**	0.25	0.12	0.16	0.09
	Closed questions**	0.20	0.10	0.10	0.06
	Open questions	0.05	0.04	0.05	0.04
	Lifestyle / psychosocial**	0.06	0.05	0.01	0.02
	Closed questions**	0.04	0.04	0.00	0.01
	Open questions**	0.02	0.03	0.00	0.01
Information-giving / counseling	Overall**	0.26	0.13	0.55	0.12
	Biomedical**	0.19	0.12	0.52	0.13
	Medical condition	0.06	0.06	0.09	0.08
	Diagnostic tests**	0.02	0.03	0.13	0.15
	Therapeutic regimen**	0.07	0.08	0.24	0.17
	others**	0.04	0.06	0.06	0.06
	Lifestyle / psychosocial*	0.07	0.09	0.03	0.05
Socioemotional	Overall**	0.43	0.11	0.29	0.08
Relationship building	Overall**	0.19	0.11	0.12	0.06
	Positive talk*	0.06	0.04	0.09	0.05
	Agreement**	0.06	0.04	0.09	0.05
	Approval	0.00	0.01	0.00	0.00
	Negative talk	0.01	0.01	0.01	0.03
	Criticism	0.00	0.01	0.01	0.03
	Disapproval	0.00	0.01	0.00	0.01
	Social conversation**	0.08	0.10	0.01	0.02
	Laughter*	0.01	0.02	0.00	0.01
	Jokes	0.00	0.01	0.00	0.00
	Chitchat**	0.03	0.09	0.01	0.01
	Emotional talk**	0.05	0.06	0.02	0.03
	Empathy*	0.01	0.01	0.00	0.01
	Concern / worry**	0.03	0.04	0.00	0.01
	Reassurance	0.01	0.03	0.01	0.02
	Legitimacy	0.00	0.00	0.00	0.01
	Self-disclosure	0.00	0.01	0.00	0.00
Partnership building	Overall**	0.24	0.09	0.16	0.09
	Verbal attentiveness	0.12	0.08	0.09	0.06
	Backchannel	0.07	0.07	0.05	0.04
	Shows understanding	0.05	0.04	0.04	0.05
	Procedural	0.05	0.04	0.04	0.04
	Giving directions	0.04	0.03	0.04	0.03
	transition**	0.02	0.02	0.00	0.01
	Facilitation**	0.07	0.05	0.04	0.04

Table 3.2 Cont.

Behavior clusters	Categories	TCM		WM	
		Mean rates	Std.	Mean rates	Std.
	Bid for repetition	0.01	0.02	0.01	0.01
	Checks**	0.05	0.04	0.02	0.03
	Asks for opinion	0.01	0.02	0.01	0.02
Missing value	Overall	0.01	0.01	0.01	0.01

Notes: *=significant at P < 0.05 level, **=significant at P < 0.01 level, N = 69

Table 3.3 Patient communication results

Behavior clusters	Categories	TCM		WM	
		Mean rates	Std.	Mean rates	Std.
Instrumental	Overall	0.63	0.14	0.57	0.10
Information seeking	Overall**	0.06	0.05	0.10	0.07
	Biomedical**	0.05	0.05	0.10	0.07
	Closed questions**	0.04	0.03	0.08	0.06
	Open questions*	0.01	0.01	0.02	0.03
	Request for service	0.01	0.02	0.01	0.02
	Lifestyle / psychosocial*	0.01	0.02	0.00	0.01
	Closed questions**	0.01	0.01	0.00	0.01
	Open questions	0.00	0.01	0.00	0.01
Information-giving	Overall**	0.57	0.14	0.47	0.13
	Biomedical	0.45	0.14	0.43	0.12
	Medical condition**	0.31	0.15	0.22	0.12
	Diagnostic tests**	0.02	0.04	0.08	0.07
	Therapeutic regimen	0.08	0.07	0.09	0.09
	others	0.03	0.05	0.04	0.05
	Lifestyle / psychosocial**	0.12	0.09	0.04	0.06
Socio-emotional	Overall	0.36	0.14	0.39	0.11
Relationship building	Overall	0.33	0.14	0.34	0.11
	Positive talk**	0.21	0.12	0.29	0.11
	Agreement**	0.21	0.12	0.29	0.11
	Approval	0.00	0.00	0.00	0.00
	Negative talk	0.00	0.01	0.00	0.01
	Criticism	0.00	0.01	0.00	0.00
	Disapproval	0.00	0.00	0.00	0.01
	Social conversation**	0.09	0.11	0.02	0.02

(*continued*)

Table 3.3 Cont.

Behavior clusters	Categories	TCM		WM	
		Mean rates	Std.	Mean rates	Std.
	Laughter*	0.02	0.02	0.00	0.01
	Chitchat**	0.08	0.10	0.02	0.02
	Emotional talk	0.02	0.03	0.03	0.05
	Empathy	0.00	0.01	0.00	0.00
	Concern / worry	0.01	0.02	0.01	0.04
	Seeking reassurance	0.00	0.01	0.01	0.02
	Legitimacy	0.00	0.00	0.00	0.01
Partnership building	Overall*	0.03	0.03	0.05	0.05
	Verbal attentiveness*	0.00	0.00	0.01	0.02
	Paraphrasing*	0.00	0.00	0.01	0.02
	Procedural	0.01	0.01	0.00	0.01
	Giving directions	0.00	0.00	0.00	0.01
	transition	0.01	0.01	0.00	0.01
	Facilitation	0.02	0.02	0.04	0.04
	Bid for repetition	0.00	0.00	0.01	0.01
	Checks	0.02	0.02	0.03	0.03
	Asks for opinion	0.00	0.00	0.00	0.01
Missing value	Overall**	0.01	0.02	0.03	0.02

Notes: *=significant at P < 0.05 level, **=significant at P < 0.01 level, N = 69

Table 3.2 shows that doctor's communication in medical encounters was mainly instrumental: in both TCM and WM, more than half of doctors' utterances (57% in TCM and 71% in WM) were instrumental, the majority of which was dedicated to data collection and information-giving and counseling. The content of the questions and information was mainly related to the biomedical domain of health-related issues, with few discussions on lifestyle and psychosocial topics. The mean number of doctors' question-asking was significantly higher in TCM than WM encounters: $F = 28.67$, $df = (4, 65)$, $p < 0.01$, $\eta^2 = 0.3$, indicating a large effect size. Yet, WM doctors provided more information to their patients than TCM doctors, $F = 87.1$, $df = (4, 65)$, $p < 0.01$, $\eta^2 = 0.57$. Compared with TCM doctors, WM doctors were more attentive to the biomedical domain of the consultation: almost all the questions initiated by WM doctors were biomedical. In addition, WM doctors provided markedly more biomedical information than TCM professionals, $F = 117.59$, $df = (4, 65)$, $p < 0.01$, $\eta^2 = 0.64$. Regarding the content of doctors' information-giving, it is clear that WM doctors were more dedicated to information-giving on diagnostic tests ($U = 328.5$, $p < 0.01$, $r = 0.4$) and therapeutic regimen ($U = 248.5$, $p < 0.01$, $r = 0.5$), but less attentive to lifestyle and psychosocial discussions ($U = 403.5$, $p < 0.05$, $r = 0.3$) than TCM doctors.

Compared to the instrumental communication, doctors' socio-emotional behavior was less observed. In both medical encounters, relational talk was least observed: 19% in TCM and 12% in WM. One difference between TCM and WM in doctors' relationship-building communication is the considerable rarity of social conversation and emotional talk in WM. Compared to the WM doctors, TCM colleagues engaged in more social conversations than WM professionals ($U = 236$, $p < 0.01$, $r = 0.6$), primarily at the level of laughs ($U = 428$, $p < 0.01$, $r = 0.4$) and nonmedical chitchat ($U = 256.5$, $p < 0.01$, $r = 0.5$). TCM doctors were also more attentive to emotional talk ($U = 288.5$, $p < 0.01$, $r = 0.5$), such as showing empathy ($U = 464$, $p < 0.05$, $r = 0.3$), and concern and worry ($U = 277.5$, $p < 0.01$, $r = 0.6$) to their patients. Compared to relationship building, doctors in this study were more attentive to partnership-building: 24% in TCM and 16% in WM of doctors' utterances function as facilitators that guide patients throughout the interaction. The major difference between TCM and WM lies in the use of transitional speech ($U = 409$, $p < 0.01$, $r = 0.3$) and utterances articulated for checking understanding ($U = 272.5$, $p < 0.01$, $r = 0.5$). Strikingly similar between TCM and WM is the scarcity of doctors' communication aimed at asking patient opinions (1%).

Patient communication showed a similarity in that it was primarily instrumental rather than socio-emotional in both encounters (Table 3.3). In both TCM and WM, patients were mainly dedicated to information-giving: 57% in TCM and 47% in WM. Yet, a closer investigation of the content of patient information suggests a discrepancy between TCM and WM encounters. There is a significantly higher observation of patient information regarding medical conditions (31% in TCM and 22% in WM, $U = 356.5$, $p < 0.01$, $r = 0.3$), and lower observation of diagnostic tests (2% in TCM and 8% in WM, $U = 290.5$, $p < 0.01$, $r = 0.4$) in TCM than in WM encounters. Another difference in patient information-giving is that TCM patients gave more lifestyle and psychosocial information than WM patients, $U = 196.5$, $p < 0.01$, $r = 0.6$. In terms of information-seeking, in general, WM patients raised more questions than TCM patients, $F = 9.56$, $df = (4, 65)$, $p < 0.01$, $\eta^2 = 0.13$. Yet, further analysis suggests that while WM patients raised more biomedical questions ($U = 339.5$, $p < 0.01$, $r = 0.4$), they were less attentive to lifestyle and psychosocial issues than TCM patients ($U = 479$, $p < 0.05$, $r = 0.2$).

Unlike doctors, patients in this study were actively engaged in relationship building (33% in TCM and 34% in WM), although most of their talk at this level was aimed at showing agreement. Patient relationship-building behavior was markedly different at the level of social conversations: more laughs ($U = 369.5$, $p < 0.01$, $r = 0.4$) and chitchat ($U = 254$, $p < 0.01$, $r = 0.5$) were observed in TCM than in WM, similar to what was observed in doctors' communication at this level. Patients' partnership-building was rare in the data, and most of the patients' utterances at this level were dedicated to checking their understanding.

3.3.2 Doctor's verbal dominance and patient-centeredness

To calculate the doctor's verbal dominance score, the total sum of doctors' utterances was divided by the total sum of patients' utterances across each

Table 3.4 Doctor–patient verbal dominance ratio

	Doctor/patient ratio	U	Sig.	Effect size
TCM	M = 0.88 (SD = 0.56)	299.5	p < 0.01	r = 0.4
WM	M = 1.11 (SD = 0.39)			

Table 3.5 Patient-centeredness score

	Patient-centeredness score	U	Sig.	Effect size
TCM	M = 1.23 (SD = 0.73)	231	p < 0.01	r = 0.5
WM	M = 0.7 (SD = 0.26)			

interaction (Roter et al., 1997). A ratio of less than one indicates that doctors were less verbally dominant and vice versa. As Table 3.4 illustrates, WM doctors were more verbally dominant than their TCM colleagues.

The patient-centeredness score (Table 3.5) was computed by dividing the total sum of psychosocial and socio-emotional statements by the total number of biomedical statements (McCarthy et al., 2013). The numerator consists of relationship building (both doctor and patient), doctors' verbal attentiveness and facilitation talk, lifestyle and psychosocial information-giving, doctors' lifestyle and psychosocial questions, and patient information-seeking. These codes describe patients' leading the conversation as well as doctors' non-instrumental behaviors in the conversation. The denominator consists of doctors' biomedical questions and information-giving, doctors' procedural talk, and patients' biomedical information-giving. This formula has been widely used in other RIAS studies (Cooper et al., 2003; Roter et al., 2008). In this study, a higher patient-centeredness ratio was reported in TCM (Mean = 1.23, SD = 0.73) than in WM consultations (Mean = 0.7, SD = 0.26), $U = 231$, $p < 0.01$, $r = 0.5$ (see Table 3.5).

3.4 Commonalities between TCM and WM

3.4.1 Doctor's dominance and patient passivity in asking questions

Earlier studies have suggested a discrepancy in participants' question-asking behavior in medical consultations. In her most widely cited work, West (1984) found that patients initiated only 9 percent of the questions in family practice resident-patient consultations. In a more recent study of a similar medical context, Pahal and Li (2006) noted that residents asked four times more questions than did patients. A higher proportion of 38.7% was reported by Ainsworth-Vaughn (2001) in her examination of oncological physician-patient encounters. In a Chinese contexts, Zhao (1999) reported that patient-initiated questions only account for 12.6% of all the questions in medical interviews. The results of this quantitative study confirmed previous findings on the interactional asymmetry between doctors and patients in medical encounters (see also Li et al., 2007; Nakayama et al., 2016; Robinson, 2003). Doctors controlled the medical interaction by asking more questions than did patients: 81% of the questions in the TCM encounter and 63% in the WM encounter were raised by the doctor. In contrast patients were quite reticent in raising questions. The disparity in participants' question-asking behavior results in an asymmetrical contribution of participants' information-giving. It seems that while doctors' major task was asking questions, patients were primarily engaged in giving information.

Patient passivity in asking questions was widely documented in earlier studies (Frankel, 1990; Roter & Frankel, 1992). In a review of intervention studies designed to encourage patient contribution to the consultation, Harrington et al. (2004) summarized that patients' question-asking represents very little of patients' verbal communication in medical interaction. Prior research has indicated that patients' information-seeking behavior may be explained by multiple factors, such as demographics (Eggly et al., 2011; Turk-Charles et al., 1997), attitudes (Wright & Frey, 2008), types of disease (Nagler et al., 2010), the doctor–patient relationship (Adamson et al., 2018), length of the visit (Dahm, 2012), and the presence of a companion (Eggly et al., 2011). Alternatively, it is likely that patients will obtain answers to some questions in the information spontaneously offered by the doctor during the course of the interaction (Roter, 1984).

Regarding the design of these questions, the current study reinforces earlier assertions that doctors frequently use closed-ended questions to limit patient response and control the flow of the discourse. In the present data, 77% of doctors' questions were closed-ended in TCM and 69% in WM encounters. Numerous studies have reported a similar observation of a preponderance of closed-ended questions in doctors' verbal contribution to the interaction (Beckman & Frankel, 1984; McCarthy et al., 2013; Ong et al., 1995; Roter & Hall, 2006; Roter & Larson, 2001). Roter and Hall (2006) argued that closed-ended questions are doctors' tools for hypothesis testing – if the hypothesis is supported, there is no need for further probing into the patient agenda, and therefore it is less time-consuming. In that sense, closed-ended questions function as doctors' information-seeking strategy: by incorporating a candidate answer (Pomerantz, 1988) into the inquiry, the doctor not only displays their knowledge and familiarity of the patient's situation but also indicates their preference for the response in terms of both content and form. In other words, the use of closed-ended questions restricts patient participation to a preferred action agenda (see Boyd & Heritage, 2006; Raymond, 2003). As Raymond (2006) noted, by formulating their inquiry to an anticipated yes/no, the doctor conveys their preference and presuppositions regarding their patients and indexes their anticipation for the best-case scenario. This understanding of closed-ended questions is supported in the present data. For example, in TCM encounters, doctors tend to ask '大便好嗎' (*Is your bowel movement regular?*). Likewise, in WM encounters, doctors frequently ask patients '胃鏡做過沒有' (*Did you have the gastroscopy examination or not?*). The TCM doctor displays their understanding that having a regular bowel movement is the best scenario. Similarly, the WM doctor suggests that having a gastroscopy examination is preferred. In both instances, the design of the question clearly favors a positive affirmation and orients the patient toward a no-problem condition. Such incorporation of preferences toward a no-problem condition is explained by Boyd and Heritage (2006) in terms of the 'principle of optimization' (p. 164). This optimization in the design of closed-ended questions somehow reflects doctors' concern for, and understanding of, the patient (Raymond, 2006). Given that patients in this study were recruited from repeated chronic encounters who have visited the same doctor several times, the overuse of closed-ended questions in doctors' verbal contribution to the interaction should be interpreted with caution. While one possible explanation is that doctors use such questions to control the patient's response, it is also likely that some interpersonal activities (e.g., showing familiarity and rapport) are performed.

Not only did doctors prefer closed-ended questions, but patients in this study also display a strong preference for closed-ended questions when seeking information from their doctors. Over 80% of patient-initiated questions were closed-ended in TCM and WM consultations. In the present data, patient-initiated questions were mainly articulated to seek advice on a range of aspects related to health. Unlike questions asked by doctors, which mainly occur in the history-taking stage (see also Boyd & Heritage, 2006), patient-initiated questions may occur in different stages. For example, in TCM encounters, patients may seek dietary advice from their doctors at conversational closings: '我蜂蜜可以吃嗎' (*Can I eat honey?*). In WM encounters, patients tend to negotiate plans for diagnostic tests or medication with the doctor: '我晚上吃降糖藥可以嗎' (*Can I take the pills that help lower the blood sugar at night?*). The findings suggest that patients overwhelmingly prefer closed-ended questions in the advice-seeking activity. While the motives of patients in using closed-ended questions are beyond the scope of this quantitative study, other studies have tried to explain such patient behaviors by doctor's topic control. For example, in a study of doctor–patient conversations in China, Luo (2015) argued that patients are more likely to use yes/no interrogatives than open-ended questions since the topics of the consultation were decided by the doctor. Here, I offer another possible explanation: given the disease conditions of the patients that require ongoing care and self-management, patients might have acquired health-related knowledge from different sources (e.g., from their earlier visits). Rather than seeking new information from the doctor, patients might take the consultation as an opportunity to confirm their understanding of how to maintain health.

3.4.2 Patients' high level of agreement

In both TCM and WM consultations, the number of times patients expressed agreement was high (21% in TCM and 29% in WM) and the number for doctors was low (6% in TCM and 9% in WM). This finding accords with Ford et al.'s (1996) study of oncological patient-clinician consultations, where 27% of patient speech and 9% of clinician speech were devoted to showing agreement. The high percentage of instances of patient agreement in the present research and the great number of doctor-initiated questions indicate that patients were attentively listening to the information and guidance offered by the doctor. Yet, the low percentage of doctor agreement and the low number of questions raised by patients suggest that patients have little opportunity to ask questions.

3.4.3 Concentration on biomedical discussions

Consistent with studies in other parts of the world (Greene & Adelman, 1996; McCarthy et al., 2013; Rost & Frankel, 1993; Roter & Larson, 2001), biomedical discussions in this study account for the majority of participants' verbal contribution to the interaction: 83% of doctor-initiated questions in TCM encounters and 96% in WM encounters were biomedical. Prior research has considered doctors' biomedical questions as an index of professional dominance and control (see Roter & Hall, 2006). Given the limited consultation time for each patient, doctors might need to make a trade-off between biomedical-intensive visits and socio-emotional visits. Doctors' lifestyle and psychosocial questions were least observed in both encounters: 6% in TCM and 1% in WM. Similarly, most of the questions initiated by patients were biomedical: 86% in TCM and 97% in WM. Regarding information-giving, the majority of doctors' (73% in TCM and 95% in WM) and patients' utterances (79% in TCM and 91% in WM) were related to the biomedical domain of information. It seems that there is a mutually aligned priority between doctors and patients to biomedical information exchange. One possible explanation is that older patients with chronic diseases tend to have a number of biomedical issues that require doctors' attention. Some patients tend to have more than one chronic condition. Prior research also suggests that older patients are more hesitant than younger patients to discuss psychosocial issues with their doctors (Greene et al., 1987; Lyness et al., 1995; Williams et al., 2007). Wittink et al. (2006, p. 308) argued that older patients are more likely to behave like a 'good patient' – one who is comfortable with the paternalistic doctor–patient relationship, respects the doctor's expertise, is compliant with the doctor's treatment recommendations, and has no negative emotional feelings. The dearth of psychosocial discussion might account for the lack of doctors' empathy and reassurance in medical consultations.

The observation of more biomedical discussions in medical encounters is also reported in other types of encounters. For example, Ford et al. (1996) found that questions related to lifestyle and psychosocial topics constituted less than a quarter of those related to biomedical issues in oncological consultations. In elderly patients' primary care, Adelman et al. (1992) noted that psychosocial talk only accounted for 11.4% of physician-raised topics and 25.7% of patient-initiated subjects.

A commonality found in both encounters is the disparity between doctors and patients in their biomedical information-seeking: while most of the biomedical questions asked by doctors were related to the medical conditions, the majority of patient-initiated questions (32% in TCM and 36% in WM) were concerned with the therapeutic regimen (e.g., treatment options, diet, and medications). This observation supports Luo's (2015) assertion that Chinese patients are most active in the treatment stage of the consultation when they are involved in discussing the treatment plans and the effectiveness of the treatment with their doctors.

3.4.4 Doctors' use of backchannels and directive statements

Backchannels were found in doctors' communication in both encounters (7% in TCM and 5% in WM). Aside from the apparent function of indicating attentiveness, backchannels also shape story-telling (Tolins & Tree, 2014). By producing a minimal reaction to the patient, the doctor displays their acceptance of the patient's extensive narration, which possibly takes multiple turns. In other words, the use of backchannels is a strategy to manage the flow of information. Yet, different from closed-ended questions, backchannels are supportive tools that encourage patient elaboration. In the current data, backchannels primarily occurred in the history-taking stage of the consultation.

In both TCM and WM encounters, doctors devoted 4% of their verbal utterances to giving directions. Further analysis of the data shows two environments where directive statements primarily occur: first, during physical examinations of the patient (e.g., '舌頭看一下' *Stick out your tongue.*). Second, the doctor offered directions regarding the next appointment, plan for medication refills, and payment methods before the patient leaves (e.g., '拿著這個去付錢拿藥' *Take this form to the cashier and then go to the dispensary.*). In both instances, the offering of directions reflects the doctor's privilege to announce or shift conversational activities. In contrast, talk of this nature was absent in patient speech. The use of directive statements could be understood as an indicator of the doctor's communication control (Peck & Conner, 2011).

3.5 Differences between TCM and WM

3.5.1 Content of questions and information-giving

The RIAS analysis of the content of participants' questions reflects a disparity between TCM and WM in terms of the content of participants' questions and information-giving. In my observation, topics on diagnostic tests were more frequently discussed in WM encounters: 25% of doctors' questions in WM and 23.6% of doctors' information-giving were related to diagnostic tests. In TCM, only 4% of doctor-initiated queries and 7.7% of doctors' information-giving addressed issues related to diagnostic tests. Yet, there was a severe shortage of lifestyle and psychosocial discussions in participants' verbal contributions to WM interactions. Compared with WM, TCM conversations include more lifestyle and psychosocial talk in participants' question-asking and information-giving.

One possible explanation of the disparity in communication related to diagnostic tests in TCM and WM is their different diagnostic approaches to disease.

As an evidence-based approach to medicine, WM heavily relies on diagnostic tests in the diagnostic process. Tests such as blood tests, a gastroscopy examination, and a colonoscopy are important tools to identify molecular changes in the human body. In the absence of previous diagnostic test reports, WM doctors usually arrange for or recommend that patients take a test before diagnosing. Therefore, utterances such as '胃鏡做過沒有' (*Did you have the gastroscopy examination or not?*) and '胃鏡在哪裡做的' (*Where did you have the gastroscopy?*) were frequently observed in WM encounters. Patients with chronic diseases were usually recommended to undergo regular diagnostic tests to monitor their health conditions. While TCM diagnosis may also rely on diagnostic test reports due to medical integration, the conventional diagnostic procedure (inspection, auscultation and olfaction, inquiry, and palpation) is still the norm that guides the doctor through the interaction. This argument may also explain two other observations in this study: first, TCM doctors asked more questions than their WM colleagues (31% in TCM and 16% in WM). Second, TCM patients gave greater verbal contributions to describing their medical conditions than did WM patients (31% in TCM and 22% in WM). TCM views the patient as a holistic entity that is 'comprised of and subject to elements and forces of nature as a whole' (Wang & Li, 2005, p. 177). Seen in this light, the physical disorder of the human body can be explained by multiple factors, ranging from molecular changes to a psychosocial crisis and lifestyle changes. Therefore, TCM doctors usually explore patient health from a range of aspects that relate to their life and health.

Participants' verbal contributions regarding biomedical therapeutic regimens were also markedly different. Doctors' information-giving on this topic in WM encounters far outnumbered that in TCM encounters. Further analysis suggests that WM patients asked more therapeutic-related questions than TCM patients (see discussion in Section 3.43).

3.5.2 Social talk and emotional alignment

WM encounters had a severe lack of social conversation and emotional talk, possibly due to participants' prime focus on biomedical discussion. There was no laughter or jokes.

Participants in TCM encounters engaged in significantly more social conversations: nearly 10% of participants' utterances were concerned with topics irrelevant to the purpose of the current visit. The greater amount of social talk in TCM encounters reflects a more relaxed medical environment and a closer doctor–patient relationship. Prior research has supported the importance of small talk in medical interactions. For example, Coupland (2000) posited that given the nature of geriatrics, discussions of family and social connections might trigger discussions of issues relevant to doctors' expertise. Walsh (2007) observed clinical interactions between speech-language pathologists and patients with communication disorders associated with stroke and chronic schizophrenia. Using discourse analysis, she considered the association between informal talk, rapport-building, and asymmetry of power relations. She argued that informal talk provides an opportunity for patients to raise their concerns in naturally occurring troubles-telling. In that sense, aside from its interpersonal functions, informal social talk apparently has therapeutic power. The greater amount of social talk in TCM encounters might be fairly explained by the philosophy of TCM. TCM considers human beings as a holistic unity and tries to understand patients based on both internal (what is wrong in the human body) and external (the outside environ-ment within which the patient interacts with the society) factors. As Penn and Watermeyer (2012) suggested, talk that seems to be aside and small can also yield critical diagnostic and therapeutic information. On the other hand, the lack of social talk in WM encounters and the number of biomedical discussions (e.g., talk concerning diagnostic tests) reflects a highly instrumental communication style.

Doctors also exhibited differences in verbalizing their concerns and empathy. In the WM data, no single concern or worry was conveyed by the doctor in 93% of the consultations recorded. The lack of doctors' emotional statements and the absence of social talk are indicators of an instrumental communication style. As Zimmermann et al. (2007) claimed, one way to discourage patients from emo-tional disclosure is to privilege biomedical discussion in consultations. It seems that WM doctors were primarily engaged in accomplishing the instrumental tasks of the consultation, being less attentive to their patients' emotional and psycho-social well-being. It is also likely that given the shorter consultation length in WM than in TCM, doctors had a restricted length of time to pursue interper-sonal tasks. Compared to WM, TCM consultations were longer. TCM doctors had more time to address both the biomedical and emotional concerns of the patient. As Eide et al. (2004) pointed out, time limits might account for the lack of emotional discussions in medical consultations. In the present study, a medium correlation was found between length of consultation and doctors' emotional talk using Cohen's (1992) guideline (r (67) = 0.3, p < 0.05).

3.5.3 Doctors' facilitating behaviors

Doctors' facilitating behaviors (i.e., behaviors that invite patient collaboration) are considered one of the five dimensions of patient-centeredness (see Mead & Bower, 2000). This study found a clinical difference in one such behavior in doctor's verbal utterances: doctors' checking of their understanding. This behavior was primarily observed after patients' information-giving. In TCM encounters, 5% of doctors' verbal utterances were produced to check understanding, compared to 2% in WM. Given that older patients might have some aging-related cognitive decline that affects their effective communication with others (Murman, 2015), such as difficulty in communicating pain symptoms (Bruckenthal et al., 2009), doctors' receptiveness to their patients' communication is particularly important in delivering care. The more frequent use of doctors' checking in TCM visits indicates that TCM doctors were attentive to achieving mutual intelligibility with their patients. I am not arguing that WM doctors were less attentive than TCM doctors in seeking a mutual understanding with their patients. It is likely that patients in WM encounters effectively and clearly presented their information to avoid misunderstandings. Alternatively, the doctor's action of checking to understand patient information proffers conversational turns to the patient. By checking to understand patient information, the doctor offers the patient an opportunity to confirm or correct what has been said (see Schegloff, 1992 for the concept of repair). In so doing, the doctor also displays their respect to the patient.

3.5.4 Communication patterns

Roter et al. (1997) described five doctor–patient communication patterns in primary care consultations: narrowly biomedical, expanded biomedical, bio-psychosocial, psychosocial, and consumerist. Roter et al. characterized these encounters based on the distribution of biomedical and psychosocial discussions, plus the number of doctor-initiated questions. In the narrowly biomedical encounter, participants' biomedical talk is almost 14 times greater than psychosocial talk. A more moderate ratio of biomedical/psychosocial talk (a threefold difference) characterizes the expanded biomedical encounter. In the bio-psychosocial encounter, participants' biomedical talk is twice as much as biomedical talk. A psychosocial encounter features an even distribution of psychosocial and biomedical talk in doctors' communication and a greater percentage of psychosocial discussions in patients' communication. The consumerist encounter features a high frequency of patient questions and doctors' information-giving.

Using Roter et al.'s criteria, a cluster analysis was performed to identify the patterns of participants' communication in both encounters. Communication clusters entered in the analysis mainly included question-asking (both biomedical and lifestyle/psychosocial) and information-giving (both biomedical and lifestyle/psychosocial). In the present study, TCM doctors' communication is expanded biomedical, with 3.4 times as much biomedical (44%) as psychosocial talk (13%). Similarly, TCM patients' communication can also be considered as expanded biomedical, with 3.8 times as much biomedical (50%) as psychosocial talk (13%). However, WM doctors' communication is narrowly biomedical with a 17-fold difference in the biomedical (68%) and psychosocial talk (4%). WM patients' communication is also narrowly biomedical, with a 13-fold difference in their biomedical (53%) and psychosocial talk (4%).

A doctor's verbal dominance score was calculated for all visits to distinguish these encounters as being doctor-directed or jointly collaborated. The scores presented in Table 3.4 show the difference between TCM and WM in relation to the doctor's verbal control and are significant ($U = 299.5$, $p < 0.01$, $r = 0.4$). The results suggest that TCM encounters feature a more collaborative communication between doctors and patients, with a ratio of less than one. Compared with TCM, WM encounters might be more doctor-directed or guided, with a percentage greater than one.

Regarding the patient-centeredness score, the ratio was 1.23 in TCM and 0.7 in WM visits. This finding gives further insight into considerations of the biomedical/psychosocial balance in both encounters. To measure patient-centeredness, the total number of psychosocial and socio-emotional utterances in both participants' communication was divided by the sum of participants' biomedical communication (see details in Section 3.32). The higher patient-centeredness score in TCM and the greater number of doctors' relationship-building and partnership-building communication in TCM (see Table 3.2) suggest that TCM encounters are more patient-centered than WM encounters. Note that the score reported in the WM sample is not extremely low compared with the values seen in the literature in other medical settings. For example, McCarthy et al. (2013) reported a value of 0.44 in emergency physicians' communication, using the same formula. Paasche-Orlow and Roter's (2003) study of internal medicine and family practice reported a value of 1.1 in physicians' communication. Compared with these studies, the current TCM sample reports a higher patient-centeredness value. However, Helitzer et al.'s (2011) study of primary care encounters reported a score of 2.42 in providers' communication. The discrepancy in the values reported in the literature is not surprising, given the differences in multiple variables such as clinical settings, participants, and seriousness of the illness.

3.6 Summary

The primary aim of this chapter has been to quantify and compare the verbal communication behaviors of doctors and older patients in TCM and WM encounters. Four main types of communication are examined: question-asking, information-giving, relationship-building, and partnership-building. Using RIAS codes, I have attempted to distinguish participants' communication at two levels: between instrumental and socio-emotional communication, and between biomedical and psychosocial communication.

The most frequent behavior that dominated all consultations is not unsurprisingly, instrumental communication (question-asking and information-giving) from both doctors and patients. Doctors, on average, ask more questions and offer more information related to the biomedical health of the patient. There are few social conversations and emotional disclosure in medical consultations. The large number of participants' instrumental communications and the low percentage of socio-emotional communications indicate that participants are primarily task-oriented.

I then proceed to discuss the differences between TCM and WM encounters concerning participants' communication patterns. Three scores are calculated: the biomedical/psychosocial ratio, the doctor's verbal dominance, and the patient-centeredness score. The three scores are then discussed based on considerations of participants' performance in specific communication activities (e.g., question-asking). WM encounters are more biomedical and doctor-directed than TCM visits in this sample, with greater doctors' verbal contribution to biomedical information-giving. In particular, information about diagnostic tests and therapeutic regimens is more frequently observed in WM doctors' communication, as might be expected given the different diagnostic approaches of the two medical approaches.

References

Adamson, M., Choi, K., Notaro, S., & Cotoc, C. (2018). The doctor–patient relationship and information-seeking behavior: Four orientations to cancer communication. *Journal of Palliative Care, 33*(2), 79–87. https://doi.org/10.1177%2F0825859718759881

Adelman, R. D., Greene, M. G., Charon, R., & Friedman, E. (1992). The content of physician and elderly patient interaction in the medical primary care encounter. *Communication Research, 19*(3), 370–380. https://doi.org/10.1177%2F009365092019003004

Ainsworth-Vaughn, N. (2001). The discourse of medical encounters. In D. Schiffrin, D. Tannen, & H. E. Hamilton (Eds.), *The handbook of discourse analysis* (pp. 453–469). Malden: Blackwell.

Beckman, H. B., & Frankel, R. M. (1984). The effect of physician behavior on the collection of data. *Annals of Internal Medicine, 101*(5), 692–696. https://doi.org/10.7326/0003-4819-101-5-692

Boyd, E., & Heritage, J. (2006). Taking the history: Questioning during comprehensive history-taking. In J. Heritage & D. W. Maynard (Eds.), *Communication in medical care: Interaction between primary care physicians and patients* (pp. 151–184). Cambridge: Cambridge University Press. https://doi.org/10.1017/CBO9780511607172.008

Bruckenthal, P., Reid, M. C., & Reisner, L. (2009). Special issues in the management of chronic pain in older patients. *Pain Medicine, 10*(S2), S67-S78. https://doi.org/10.1111/j.1526-4637.2009.00667.x

Chui, K. (1996). Organization of repair in Chinese conversation. *Text, 16*(3), 343–372. https://doi.org/10.1515/text.1.1996.16.3.343

Cohen, J. (1992). A power primer. *Psychological Bulletin, 112*(1), 155–159. https://psycnet.apa.org/doi/10.1037/0033-2909.112.1.155

Cooper, L. A., Roter, D. L., Johnson, R. L., Ford, D. E., Steinwachs, D. M., & Powe, N. R. (2003). Patient-centered communication, ratings of care, and concordance of patient and physician race. *Annals of Internal Medicine, 139*(11), 907–915. https://doi.org/10.7326/0003-4819-139-11-200312020-00009

Coupland, J. (2000). Introduction: Sociolinguistic perspectives on small talk. In J. Coupland (Ed.), *Small talk* (pp. 1–25). London: Pearson Education.

Coupland, J., Coupland, N., & Robinson, J. D. (1992). 'How are you?': Negotiating phatic communion. *Language in Society, 21*(2), 207–230. https://doi.org/10.1017/S0047404500015268

Dahm, M. R. (2012). Tales of time, terms and patient information-seeking behavior – An exploratory qualitative study. *Health Communication, 27*(7), 682–689. https://doi.org/10.1080/10410236.2011.629411

Eggly, S., Harper, F. W. K., Penner, L. A., Gleason, M. J., Foster, T., & Albrecht, T. L. (2011). Variation in question asking during cancer clinical interactions: A potential source of disparities in access to information. *Patient Education and Counseling, 82*(1), 63–68. https://doi.org/10.1016/j.pec.2010.04.008

Eide, H., Quera, V., Graugaard, P., & Finset, A. (2004). Physician–patient dialogue surrounding patients' expression of concern: Applying sequence analysis to RIAS. *Social Science & Medicine, 59*(1), 145–155. https://doi.org/10.1016/j.socscimed.2003.10.011

Ford, S., Fallowfield, L., & Lewis, S. (1996). Doctor–patient interactions in oncology. *Social Science and Medicine, 42*(11), 1511–1519. https://doi.org/10.1016/0277-9536(95)00265-0

Frankel, R. M. (1990). Talking in interviews: A dispreference for patient-initiated questions. In G. Psathas (Ed.), *Interaction competence* (pp. 231–61). Lanham, MD: University Press of America.

Greene, M. G., & Adelman, R. (1996). Psychosocial factors in older patients' medical encounters. *Research on Aging, 18*(1), 84–102. https://doi.org/10.1177%2F0 164027596181006

Greene, M. G., Hoffman, S., Charon, R., & Adelman, R. (1987). Psychosocial concerns in the medical encounter: A comparison of the interactions of doctors with their old and young patients. *The Gerontologist, 27*(2), 164–168. https://doi.org/10.1093/geront/ 27.2.164

Harrington, J., Noble, L. M., & Newman, S. P. (2004). Improving patients' communication with doctors: A systematic review of intervention studies. *Patient Education and Counseling, 52*(1), 7–16. https://doi.org/10.1016/S0738-3991(03)00017-X

Hayashi, R. (1991). Floor structure of English and Japanese conversation. *Journal of Pragmatics, 16*(1), 1–30. https://doi.org/10.1016/0378-2166(91)90003-G

Helitzer, D. L., LaNoue, M., Wilson, B., de Hernandez, B. U., Warner, T., & Roter, D. (2011). A randomized controlled trial of communication training with primary care providers to improve patient-centeredness and health risk communication. *Patient Education and Counseling, 82*(1), 21–29. https://doi.org/10.1016/j.pec. 2010.01.021

Holmes, J. (2000). Doing collegiality and keeping control at work: Small talk in government departments. In J. Coupland (Ed.), *Small talk* (pp. 32–61). London: Pearson Education.

Li, H. Z., Koehn, C., Desroches, N. G., Yum, Y-O., & Deagle, G. (2007). Asymmetrical talk between physicians and patients: A quantitative discourse analysis. *Canadian Journal of Communication, 32*(3), 417–433. https://doi.org/10.22230/cjc.2007v32n3a1959

Luo, X. (2015). Patients' interrogative choices in Chinese doctor–patient conversations. *Studies in Sociology of Science, 6*(4), 65–69. http://dx.doi.org/10.3968/n

Lyness, J. M., Cox, C., Curry, J., Conwell, Y., King, D. A., & Caine, E. D. (1995). Older age and the underreporting of depressive symptoms. *Journal of the American Geriatrics Society, 43*(3), 216–221. https://doi.org/10.1111/j.1532-5415.1995.tb07325.x

McCarthy, D. M., Buckley, B. A., Engel, K. G., Forth, V. E., Adams, J. G., & Cameron, K. A. (2013). Understanding patient-provider conversations: What are we talking about?. *Academic Emergency Medicine, 20*(5), 441–448. https://doi.org/10.1111/ acem.12138

Mead, N., & Bower, P. (2000). Patient-centeredness: A conceptual framework and review of the empirical literature. *Social Science & Medicine, 51*(7), 1087–1110. https://doi. org/10.1016/S0277-9536(00)00098-8

Murman, D. L. (2015). The impact of aging on cognition. *Seminars in Hearing, 36*(3), 111–121. https://dx.doi.org/10.1055%2Fs-0035-1555115

Nagler, R. H., Gray, S. W., Romantan, A., Kelly, B. J., Demichele, A., Armstrong, K., Schwartz, J. S., & Hornik, R. C. (2010). Differences in information seeking among breast, prostate, and colorectal cancer patients: Results from a population-based survey. *Patient Education and Counseling, 81*(S1), s54-s62. https://doi.org/10.1016/j.pec. 2010.09.010

Nakayama, C., Kimata, S., Oshima, T., Kato, A., & Nitta, A. (2016). Analysis of pharmacist-patient communication using the Roter Method of Interaction Process Analysis System. *Administrative Pharmacy, 12*(2), 319–326. https://doi.org/10.1016/j.sapharm. 2015.05.007

Ong, L. M. L., De Haes, J. C. J. M., Hoos, A. M., & Lammes, F. B. (1995). Doctor–patient communication: A review of the literature. *Social Science & Medicine, 40*(7), 903–918. https://doi.org/10.1016/0277-9536(94)00155-M

Paasche-Orlow, M. & Roter, D. (2003). The communication patterns of internal medicine and family practice physicians. *Journal of the American Board of Family Practice, 16*(6), 485–493. https://doi.org/10.3122/jabfm.16.6.485

Pahal, J. S., & Li, H. Z. (2006). The dynamics of resident-patient communication: Data from Canada. Communication & *Medicine, 3*(2), 161–170. https://doi.org/10.1515/cam.2006.018

Peck, B. M., & Conner, S. (2011). Talking with me or talking at me? The impact of status characteristics on doctor–patient interaction. *Sociological Perspectives, 54*(4), 547–567. https://doi.org/10.1525%2Fsop.2011.54.4.547

Penn, C., & Watermeyer, J. (2012). When asides become central: Small talk and big talk in interpreted health interactions. *Patient Education and Counseling, 88*(3), 391–398. https://doi.org/10.1016/j.pec.2012.06.016

Pomerantz, A. (1988). Offering a candidate answer: An information-seeking strategy. *Communication Monographs, 55*(4), 360–373. https://psycnet.apa.org/doi/10.1080/03637758809376177

Ragan, S. L. (2000). Sociable talk in women's health care contexts: Two forms of non-medical talk. In J. Coupland (Ed.), *Small talk* (pp. 269–287). London: Pearson Education. http://dx.doi.org/10.4324/9781315838328-15

Raymond, G. (2003). Grammar and social organization: Yes/no interrogatives and the structure of responding. *American Sociological Review, 68*(6), 939-967. https://psycnet.apa.org/doi/10.2307/1519752

Raymond, G. (2006). Questions at work: Yes/no type interrogatives in institutional contexts. In P. Drew, G. Raymond, & D. Weinberg (Eds.), *Talk and interaction in social research methods* (pp. 122–140). London: Sage. https://dx.doi.org/10.4135/9781849209991.n8

Robinson, J. D. (2003). An interactional structure of medical activities during acute visits and its implications for patients' participation. *Health Communication, 15*(1), 27–57. https://doi.org/10.1207/S15327027HC1501_2

Rost, K., & Frankel, R. (1993). The introduction of the older patients' problems in medical visit. *Journal of Health and Aging, 5*(3), 387–401. https://doi.org/10.1177/089826439300500306

Roter, D. L. (1977). *The Roter method of interaction process analysis (RIAS manual).* Baltimore: Johns Hopkins University Press.

Roter, D. L. (1984). Patient questions asking in physician-patient interaction. *Health Psychology, 3*(5), 395–409.

Roter, D. L., & Frankel, R. (1992). Quantitative and qualitative approaches to the evaluation of the medical dialogue. *Social Science & Medicine, 34*(10), 1097–1103. https://doi.org/10.1016/0277-9536(92)90283-V

Roter, D. L., & Hall, J. A. (2004). Physician gender and patient-centered communication: A critical review of empirical research. *Annual Review of Public Health, 25*, 497–519. https://doi.org/10.1146/annurev.publhealth.25.101802.123134

Roter, D. L., & Hall, J. A. (2006). *Doctors talking with patients / patients talking with doctors: Improving communication in medical visits.* Westport: Praeger.

Roter, D. L., Hall, J. A., & Katz, N. R. (1987). Relations between physicians' behaviors and analogue patients' satisfaction, recall, and impressions. *Medical Care, 25*(5), 437–451. https://psycnet.apa.org/doi/10.1097/00005650-198705000-00007

Roter, D. L., & Larson, S. (2001). The relationship between residents' and attending physicians' communication during primary care visits: An illustrative use of the Roter Interaction Analysis System. *Health Communication, 13*(1), 33–48. https://doi.org/10.1207/S15327027HC1301_04

Roter, D. L., & Larson, S. (2002). The Roter interaction analysis system (RIAS): Utility and flexibility for analysis of medical interactions. *Patient Education and Counseling, 46*(4), 243–251. https://doi.org/10.1016/S0738-3991(02)00012-5

Roter, D. L., Larson, S. M., Beach, M. C., & Cooper, L. A. (2008). Interactive and evaluative correlates of dialogue sequence: A simulation study applying the RIAS to turn taking structures. *Patient Education and Counseling, 71*(1), 26–33. https://doi.org/10.1016/j.pec.2007.10.019

Roter, D. L., Stewart, M., Putnam, S. M., Lipkin, M., Stiles, W. B., & Inui, T. S. (1997). Communication patterns of primary care physicians. *JAMA, 277*(4), 350–356.

Schegloff, E. A. (1992). Repair after next turn: The last structurally provided defense of intersubjectivity in conversation. *American Journal of Sociology, 97*(5), 1295–1345. https://doi.org/10.1086/229903

Schegloff, E. A., & Sacks, H. (1973). Opening up closings. *Semiotica, 8*, 289–327. https://doi.org/10.1515/semi.1973.8.4.289

Tolins, J., & Tree, J. E. F. (2014). Addressee backchannels steer narrative development. *Journal of Pragmatics, 70*, 152–164. https://doi.org/10.1016/j.pragma.2014.06.006

Turk-Charles, S., Meyerowitz, B. E., & Gatz, M. (1997). Age differences in information-seeking among cancer patients. *Internal Journal of Aging and Human Development, 45*(2), 85–98. https://doi.org/10.2190%2F7CBT-12K3-GA8H-F68R

Walsh, I. P. (2007). Small talk is 'big talk' in clinical discourse: Appreciating the value of conversation in SLP clinical interactions. *Topics in Language Disorders, 27*(1), 24–36. http://dx.doi.org/10.1097/00011363-200701000-00004

Wang, S. B., & Li, Y. M. (2005). Traditional Chinese medicine. In O. Devinsky, S. V. Pacia & S. C. Shachter (Eds.), *Complementary and alternative therapies for epilepsy* (pp. 177–182). New York: Demos Medical Publishing.

West, C. (1984). *Routine complications: Troubles with talk between doctors and patients.* Bloomington: Indiana University Press.

Williams, S. L., Haskard, K. B., & DiMatteo, M. R. (2007). The therapeutic effects of the physician-older patient relationship: Effective communication with vulnerable older patients. *Clinical Interventions in Aging, 2*(3), 453–467.

Wittink, M. N., Barg, F. K., & Gallo, J. J. (2006). Unwritten rules of talking to doctors about depression: Integrating qualitative and quantitative methods. *Annals of Family Medicine, 4*(4), 302–309. https://doi.org/10.1370/afm.558

Wright, K. B., & Frey, L. R. (2008). Communication and care in an acute cancer center: The effects of patients' willingness to communicate about health, health-care environment perceptions, and health status on information seeking, participation in care practices, and satisfaction. *Health Communication, 23*(4), 369–379. https://doi.org/10.1080/10410230802229886

Zhao, B. (1999). Asymmetry and mitigation in Chinese medical interviews. *Health Communication, 11*(3), 209–214. https://doi.org/10.1207/S15327027HC110303

Zimmermann, C., Piccolo, L. D., & Finset, A. (2007). Cues and concerns by patients in medical consultations: A literature review. *Psychological Bulletin, 133*(3), 438–463. https://doi.org/10.1037/0033-2909.133.3.438

4 Patient evaluation and satisfaction

4.1 Understanding patient satisfaction

Numerous studies have indicated patient satisfaction might be influenced by multiple variables. Apart from health-related concerns (i.e., outcomes), patient satisfaction is also predicted by factors relating to patient characteristics (e.g., age, gender, and health status), doctors' communication styles, and some organizational factors (e.g., visit length). Given the purpose of this research, I will focus on the association between doctors' communication and patient satisfaction.

Prior research has suggested that patient satisfaction can be predicted by professionals' communication styles and many scholars advocate a PCC style that includes attentive listening (Baker et al., 2020), immediacy (Wanzer et al., 2004), the use of open- and closed-ended questions (Ishikawa et al., 2002), shared decision-making (Stewart, 2001), showing empathy (Kim et al., 2004), giving voice to patients' lifeworld issues (Barry et al., 2001), and engaging in small talk (Penn & Watermeyer, 2012). These behaviors show doctors' attitudes toward treating the patient as a whole person rather than a case. Professionals' patient-centered behaviors are particularly crucial in managing older patients with multiple chronic conditions because this population needs long-term care and is more psychologically dependent on their social connections, such as families, friends, and doctors. Reviews of the literature that reports on the positive association between professionals' communication competence and older patients' satisfaction are quite accessible (Finkelstein et al., 2017; Greene & Adelman, 2001; Greene et al., 1994). A consistent finding of these studies is that older patients prefer encounters in which they are encouraged (e.g., doctors' use of open-ended questions and attentive listening), supported (e.g., emotional display), and not rushed.

While PCC includes behaviors in the instrumental and affective domain of communication, there is growing evidence that patient satisfaction is reflected more clearly by affective and relational communication than instrumental communication (Epstein & Street, 2007). For example, in a meta-analysis of cancer patients' communication and physician behaviors, Venetis et al. (2009) found that instrumental communication (e.g., question-asking and information-giving) is less strongly associated with satisfaction than PCC. The authors operationalized

DOI: 10.4324/9781003161929-4

PCC to that which attends to patients' affective needs, values, preferences, and patient empowerment; and defined patient-centered behaviors to include participants' affective and participation behaviors (physicians' prompting for patient involvement and patients' question-asking). In an earlier study, in the 1970s, Ben-Sira (1976) highlighted the importance of professionals' affective communication in influencing patient satisfaction. As Ben-Sira indicated, since patients are not equipped with the esoteric knowledge and expertise to evaluate professionals' instrumental skills, their evaluation of the medical encounter largely depends on their assessment of doctors' affective communication (see also Hong & Oh, 2019). In a series of studies of GP consultations, Ben-Sira (1980, 1982) further developed this argument and demonstrated the crucial role of physicians' affective communication in evaluating professional competence. Likewise, Hesse and Rauscher (2018) examined the role of affectionate communication and patient outcomes. They found that affectionate communication is strongly associated with patient satisfaction, while affection deprivation negatively relates to satisfaction.

Drawing from insights gained from earlier research, the quantitative study here focuses on patient perceptions of their doctor's communication performance in the relational domain of communication. The three research questions are:

(1) How do patients rate their doctors' communication performance in different medical encounters?
(2) Are patients satisfied with the overall medical interaction?
(3) Do patient evaluations of doctors' communication performance correlate with their satisfaction with the overall medical interaction?

4.2 Relational communication scale

This study used the 14-item RCS (Burgoon et al., 1987) to assess the following information:

(1) Demographic data regarding age, gender, type of practice, and the number of visits prior to the current interaction.
(2) Evaluations of doctors' communication competencies over 14 items. Items are fielded into six domains of relational communication: immediacy, similarity, receptivity, composure, formality, dominance and equality. Patients were asked to indicate the degree of agreement to 14 statements using a 5-point Likert scale that ranged from 'strongly agree' to 'strongly disagree.
(3) Global patient satisfaction with the medical encounter. Patients were asked to indicate the degree of satisfaction using a 5-point Likert scale that ranged from 'very satisfied' to 'very dissatisfied'.

The immediacy scale attempts to address issues of professional involvement and doctor–patient intimacy. The similarity scale reflects doctor–patient alignment to values and attitudes. The receptivity scale measures rapport and openness. The composure scale provides messages on doctors' ways of communication, examining expressions such as relaxation, anger, and anxiety. The formality scale assesses the extent to which medical communication is formal or informal. Finally, the dominance scale examines patient perceptions about the various degree of conversational equality, control, and power relations (see Burgoon & Le Poire, 1999).

Items with negative wording were reverse scored. After reverse scoring for the 14 items among 45 patients, the reliability was acceptable ($\alpha = 0.78$). Content validity was based on whether items correlate significantly. Spearman's rho tests showed significant correlations across the six dimensions at a significance level of $p < 0.05$. All dimensions were significantly associated with global satisfaction. In the main study, the reliability after reverse scoring among 69 patients was acceptable ($\alpha = 0.7$). Patient agreement with positively worded items was translated to satisfied (agree) and very satisfied (strongly agree). Patient agreement with negatively worded items was translated to dissatisfied and very dissatisfied.

Participants' responses were collected immediately after their medical consultations to maximize patient recall (Neuman, 2011). In accordance with the patient's request, survey questions were read to the patient. One explanation for this unusual way of collecting questionnaire data is that the patients in this study are older adults who might have challenges in paper reading due to age-related sight loss. Patients were also encouraged to elaborate on any of the survey items. Patient comments were structured and recorded on the margin of the questionnaire.

The questionnaire was pretested for completeness and clarity by 45 older adults. Using a Chinese version of the RCS-14 (Wang, 2010), all patients understood the questions with no difficulty. Shapiro-Wilk tests were used to assess the normality. With the null hypothesis being rejected (w = 0.87 for similarity, 0.95 for receptivity, 0.94 for immediacy, 0.93 for composure, 0.59 for formality, 0.9 for dominance, and 0.78 for global satisfaction), comparisons of patient evaluations and global satisfaction in TCM and WM were analyzed via the Mann-Whitney U test.

4.3 Results

Patients who participated in the RIAS study also participated in the survey. Table 4.1 summarizes the demographic and practice characteristics of the 69 older adults who responded to the survey.

None of the patients were initial visitors. Nearly 61% of the patients had visited the same doctor at least four times. There was no marked difference regarding the number of respondents in terms of age and practice types.

Figure 4.1 presents the item correlation of the survey. Items on similarity and receptivity were significantly correlated with items on each of the other domains. Yet, items on immediacy, formality, and dominance were related to items on each of the other domains except composure. The magnitude of the effect size for associations between these items ranged from medium to large ($-0.323 \leq r_s (67) \leq 0.853$).

Table 4.1 Demographic and practice characteristics of patients

Gender	
Male	32
Female	37
Age	
Mean	63
Standard deviation	8.5
Minimum	50
Maximum	82
Practice	
TCM	30
WM	39
Number of prior visits	
1	3
2	12
3	12
More than 4	42

Correlations

			immediacy	similarity	receptivity	composure	formality	dominance	satisfaction
Spearman's rho	immediacy	Correlation Coefficient	1.000	.656**	.853**	.187	-.617**	-.540**	.744**
		Sig. (2-tailed)		.000	.000	.124	.000	.000	.000
		N	69	69	69	69	69	69	69
	similarity	Correlation Coefficient	.656**	1.000	.729**	.248*	-.571**	-.323**	.585**
		Sig. (2-tailed)	.000		.000	.040	.000	.007	.000
		N	69	69	69	69	69	69	69
	receptivity	Correlation Coefficient	.853**	.729**	1.000	.260*	-.683**	-.474**	.735**
		Sig. (2-tailed)	.000	.000		.031	.000	.000	.000
		N	69	69	69	69	69	69	69
	composure	Correlation Coefficient	.187	.248*	.260*	1.000	.022	-.103	.170
		Sig. (2-tailed)	.124	.040	.031		.861	.400	.162
		N	69	69	69	69	69	69	69
	formality	Correlation Coefficient	-.617**	-.571**	-.683**	.022	1.000	.365**	-.622**
		Sig. (2-tailed)	.000	.000	.000	.861		.002	.000
		N	69	69	69	69	69	69	69
	dominance	Correlation Coefficient	-.540**	-.323**	-.474**	-.103	.365**	1.000	-.382**
		Sig. (2-tailed)	.000	.007	.000	.400	.002		.001
		N	69	69	69	69	69	69	69
	satisfaction	Correlation Coefficient	.744**	.585**	.735**	.170	-.622**	-.382**	1.000
		Sig. (2-tailed)	.000	.000	.000	.162	.000	.001	
		N	69	69	69	69	69	69	69

**. Correlation is significant at the 0.01 level (2-tailed).

*. Correlation is significant at the 0.05 level (2-tailed).

Note duplicates above and below the diagonal

Figure 4.1 Survey item correlations.

All the six relational domains of doctors' communication except composure were markedly correlated to global satisfaction, with a medium to large magnitude of effect size ($-0.382 \leq r_s (67) \leq 0.744$). Doctors' immediacy, similarity, and receptivity were positively related to global satisfaction, while dominance and formality were negatively associated with global satisfaction. Among all

Table 4.2 Practice-related differences in patient satisfaction

	Immediacy	*Similarity*	*Receptivity*	*Composure*	*Formality*	*Dominance*	*Global*
Mean rank							
TCM	16	21.08	16.95	31.6	48.15	46.38	17.83
WM	49.62	45.71	48.88	37.62	24.88	26.24	48.21
Sig.	0.00*	0.00*	0.00*	0.21	0.00*	0.00*	0.00*
Z	−7.01	−5.4	−6.66	−1.26	−5.92	−4.41	−0.71
R	−0.84	−0.65	−0.8		−0.71	−0.53	−0.84

Notes: *=significant at P < 0.01 level, N = 69.

the relational domains, immediacy ($r_s = 0.744$) and 'receptivity' ($r_s = 0.735$) were most strongly related to global satisfaction.

Table 4.2 shows the practice-related differences in patient satisfaction on the survey items, using the Mann-Whitney U test. Differences in patients' evaluation were observed across all the six domains of relational communication except composure, with medium to large effect size. The items having to do with immediacy and receptivity showed the biggest differences. These results suggest that on each of the five relational aspects (immediacy, similarity, receptivity, formality, and dominance), TCM doctors received greater patient satisfaction than their WM colleagues. Patients' global satisfaction with their medical encounters was significantly higher in TCM than in WM visits ($p < 0.01$, $Z = -7.01$, $r = -0.84$). An independent sample *t*-test was used to calculate the mean scores and standard deviations of global satisfaction. The mean scores of global satisfaction were 1.9 (SD = 0.25) in TCM and 2.9 (SD = 0.42) in WM. The reported high association between relational items and global satisfaction provides evidence to support the assumption that patient satisfaction of their medical encounters can be predicted by their evaluations of doctors' affective communication.

Table 4.3 presents the practice-related mean differences on each item of the short form RCS-14. Of the 14 items, the item on attentiveness listening (item 6) shows the largest difference with a mean difference of 1.77. There were considerable differences in patient perceptions of doctors' involvement (item 1), communication of warmth (item 3), openness to patients' concerns (item 7), persuasive intent (item 12), and interest in talking with the patient (item 5). Minimal differences were observed in patient perceptions of whether doctors were relaxed in the consultation (items 8–10).

4.4 Discussion

The six domains of relational communication reflected in the RCS-14 examined patient evaluations of doctors' communication performance at a more

Table 4.3 Mean differences on RCS-14

	TCM		WM	
	Mean	*SD*	*Mean*	*SD*
Immediacy				
Item 1(+)	2.33	0.71	3.74	0.59
Item 2 (+)	2.8	0.48	2.92	0.35
Item 3 (-)	3.83	0.46	2.23	0.48
Similarity				
Item 4 (+)	2.77	0.68	3.82	0.64
Receptivity				
Item 5 (+)	2.43	0.82	3.49	0.68
Item 6 (+)	1.87	0.43	3.64	0.63
Item 7 (+)	2	0.45	3.23	0.81
Composure				
Item 8 (-)	4.1	0.76	4.08	0.87
Item 9 (+)	1.97	0.49	2.08	0.77
Item 10 (+)	2.17	0.38	2.54	0.51
Formality				
Item 11 (+)	2.7	0.47	2.03	0.16
Dominance				
Item 12 (+)	3.13	0.43	2.05	0.22
Item 13 (-)	2.67	0.48	3.64	0.54
Item 14 (+)	2.03	0.41	2.92	0.9

Note: (+) indicates positive wording and (-) indicates negative wording

interpersonal than instrumental/technical level. Consistent with prior research (Ben-Sira, 1980; Kim et al., 2004; Venetis et al., 2009), this study confirms a large and significant association between patient perceptions about doctors' relational communication and satisfaction with the medical encounter. Patient response on the survey items indicates different communication styles or modes of interaction in TCM and WM: immediacy and distance, similarity and dissimilarity, receptivity and non-receptivity, formality and informality, and dominance and equality.

Of the relational domains of communication, the immediacy construct reflects the intimacy and emotional distance between conversational partners in the interaction (see Burgoon & Hale, 1984). Immediacy behaviors indicate participants' willingness to communicate (Mehrabian, 1969), and convey warmth and closeness (Zimmerman, 1993). A review of the literature suggests that research on professionals' immediacy in medical interactions primarily focuses on nonverbal behaviors. This convention might be inspired by the work of Mehrabian (1969), where immediacy was defined as behaviors that 'enhance closeness to and nonverbal interaction with another' (p. 203). Mehrabian described several nonverbal behaviors of immediacy, such as touching, forward lean, eye contact, and body orientation. Conlee et al. (1993), in their study of physician nonverbal immediacy and patient satisfaction, reported a significant positive association between patient satisfaction and patient perceptions of the physician's immediacy. While the subjects in Conlee et al.'s study were students, Richmond et al. (2001) observed adult patients and reported similar findings. While these studies focus primarily on patient satisfaction, Ellis et al. (2016), in their review of studies on immediacy in social relational research, found that immediate behaviors could invoke participants' information-sharing, trust, attentiveness in interaction, and emotional alignment – features of a PCC encounter. In the present study, patient perceptions of doctors' immediacy behaviors were addressed by three themes: intensity of involvement (item 1), emotional arousal (item 2), and communication of warmth (item 3). On all three items, patients indicated better performance by doctors in TCM encounters and displayed greater satisfaction with TCM doctors' communication. As the most strongly related construct to the overall satisfaction ($p < 0.01$, $r = 0.744$), the finding confirms the predictive power of immediacy in assessing patient satisfaction.

The similarity construct was positively and largely associated with immediacy. It examines the extent to which patients feel that they have shared attitudes, beliefs, experiences, and personal characteristics with their doctors (Burgoon & Hale, 1984). In other words, central here is the concept of doctor–patient congruence. Prior research has indicated that patients are more satisfied when they have shared beliefs and attitudes with their doctors on different facets of communication, for example, patient participation (Jahng et al., 2005), information-sharing and power relations (Cvengros et al., 2007), and communication styles (see Watson & Gallois, 1999 for communication accommodation and patient satisfaction). Given the differences in personal likes and dislikes (e.g., some patients prefer the traditional paternalistic encounter, while others prefer a more patient-centered encounter), central here is the match between participants' attitudes, beliefs, and values. As Cousin et al. (2012) suggested in their study of physician caring and patient satisfaction, the inconsistencies in the literature on the impact of doctors' behaviors on patient satisfaction can be explained by doctor–patient disconcordance. In the current study, it is clear that doctor–patient concordance is higher in TCM than in WM visits, with greater patient satisfaction with TCM doctors in the similarity construct.

According to Burgoon and Hale (1984), the receptivity construct reflects doctors' degree of interest (item 5), attentiveness (item 6), and openness (item 7). This construct was largely and significantly associated with immediacy and similarity. Levenstein et al. (1986) argued that the doctor's receptivity to patient-provided cues is central to patient-centered care. The failure to take up these cues may result in an insufficient understanding of patients' illnesses. Across the three items of the receptivity construct, patients indicated better performance of TCM doctors than WM doctors. Interestingly, many patients explicitly pointed out that WM doctors seldom listen to their concerns:

P 26 (WM):　感覺醫生質量不行，全是檢查，說話也不聽 。('I feel that the doctor is not well qualified. It was all about diagnostic tests. The doctor did not pay attention to what I said.')

P 59 (WM):   人太多了，醫生沒法仔細聽我說話。('There are too many people. The doctor could not listen to me carefully.')

P 61 (WM):   醫生沒空聽我說話，都聽他的。('The doctor had no time to listen to me. Anything he said.')

Extensive literature has documented the importance of doctors' listening skills to patient outcomes (Anderson et al., 2007; Henry et al., 2012; Sherrill et al., 2020). Wu and Tang (2021) argued, in their study of patient satisfaction in pediatric care encounters, that a pediatrician showing attentive listening is especially appreciated in China, particularly when they have a large number of patients to visit. Wu and Tang's observation was supported in this study: while some patients displayed an understanding of their doctor's failure to listen to the patient's concerns given the number of patients to be seen, other patients cast doubt on the 'quality' of the doctor.

The formality construct was most strongly but negatively correlated with receptivity. The more satisfied patients felt with their doctors' receptivity behaviors, the less formal they perceived the encounter. Formality was positively associated with dominance. These findings have several implications: first, patients' perceptions of a formal medical encounter are featured by doctors' non-receptive behaviors such as failure to listen to the patient, lack of interest in talking with the patient, and not attending to the patient's concerns. Second, since doctors' receptivity could encourage patient participation in the medical interaction, the negative association between formality and receptivity indicates that the more patients participated in their medical consultations, the less formal the encounter and the lower the degree of professional dominance they perceive. In this study, patients reported lower formality in TCM encounters. One possible explanation is the inclusion of too many diagnostic tests in WM encounters. In contrast, TCM diagnosis was made based on both diagnostic tests and the four-step procedure (inspection, auscultation and olfaction, inquiry, and palpation). As some patients indicated:

P 63 (WM):   直接開報告，應付了事 ('They just sent you to do the diagnostic tests, so scripted and careless.')

P 26 (WM):   感覺醫生質量不行，全是檢查，說話也不聽 。('I feel that the doctor is not well qualified. It was all about diagnostic tests. The doctor did not pay attention to what I said.')

The dominance construct was negatively associated with all the other constructs of RCS-14 except formality. According to Burgoon and Hale (1984, 1987), the dominance construct seeks to describe features of persuasive (item 12) and influential intents (item 13) and power relations (item 14). While the literature seems to be inconsistent regarding the impact of professional dominance on patient satisfaction, depending on multiple variables such as patient demographics, medical contexts, and seriousness of the medical conditions, this study finds that doctors' dominance has a negative impact on the patient's appraisal of the overall medical encounter, as evidenced by the negative association between the dominance con-struct and global satisfaction (Figure 4.1). The dominance scale was most strongly but negatively associated with doctors' nonverbal immediacy, which is not unex-pected. While the immediacy scale reflects patient perceptions of doctor–patient relational intimacy, the dominance scale attends to a skewed power relation.

Interestingly, doctors' dominance was ranked lowest among the five constructs significantly associated with patient satisfaction, with a moderate effect size ($p < 0.01$, $r = -0.382$). This observation might suggest that doctors' domin-ance was considered less critical among Chinese patients than other relational behaviors. One possible explanation is that medical encounters in China feature professional dominance (Cong, 2004; Pun et al., 2018; Tu et al., 2019; Wang, 2010). In other words, professional dominance has become a norm in Chinese medical consultations. It is also likely that power relations, control, and egali-tarian relationships are less of a concern to older patients than other communi-cation behaviors (see Greene et al., 1994). In addition, the study also furthers prior knowledge by showing greater professional dominance in WM than TCM encounters.

According to Burgoon and Hale (1984), the composure construct addresses doctors' degree of tension (item 8), calmness (item 9), and relaxation (item 10). Earlier studies have indicated that professionals' composure was strongly associated with patient satisfaction (see Hall et al., 1981; Inui et al., 1982). Elsewhere, Burgoon and Hale (1987) assumed that composure is more interrelated with other relational domains than other constructs. However, the findings reported here were ad hoc in relation to earlier observations and assumptions. First, com-posure is the only construct that was not statistically correlated with patients' global satisfaction. Second, patient perceptions of doctors' composure were mod-erately associated with only two other themes: doctor-patient similarity ($p = 0.04$, $r = 0.249$) and doctors' receptivity ($p = 0.03$, $r = 0.26$), with a small effect size. One possible explanation is that the patient respondents indicated no difference in doctors' composure between TCM and WM visits (see Tables 4.2 and 4.3). This explanation might also account for the lack of association between doctors' composure and global satisfaction.

Communication reflected in these constructs/domains of relational com-munication indicates doctors' communication styles: patient-centered or doctor-dominant. While differences were observed in patient response, none of the observations should be read independently. Given the item correlations, differences in each domain of relational communication could be explained by the differences in other domains, and together, these differences result in a dis-parity in patients' overall satisfaction with the medical encounter.

4.5 Summary

This chapter has focused on patients' evaluations of their doctors' relational com-munication across six domains: immediacy, similarity, receptivity, composure, formality, and dominance. Higher patient evaluations of doctors' relational communication were reported in all the domains except composure, suggesting a more PCC style in TCM encounters than WM. The study also examines the correlation between patients' perceptions of doctors' relational communication and patients' global satisfaction with the medical encounter. Consistent with prior research on the impact of doctors' communication styles and patient satisfaction (Ben-Sira, 1980; Kim et al., 2004; Venetis et al., 2009), this study finds that doctors' PCC style and affective behaviors were largely and significantly associated with patients' overall satisfaction with the medical encounter. Conversely, a doctor-centered style with behaviors indicating dominance and formality was negatively related to patient satisfaction. However, different from prior observations (Hall et al., 1981), doctors' composure was not robust in explaining the variations in patient satisfaction in the sample population.

References

Anderson, R., Barbara, A., & Fieldman, S. (2007). What patients want: A content analysis of key qualities that influence patient satisfaction. *Medical Practice Management, 22*(5), 255–261.

Baker, S. C., Watson, B. M., Jamieson, B., & Jamieson, R. (2020). How do patients define satisfaction? The role of patient perceptions of their participation and health provider emotional expression. *Health Communication, 36*(14), 1970–1979. https://doi.org/10.1080/10410236.2020.1808409

Barry, C. A., Stevenson, F. A., Britten, N., Barber, N., & Bradley, C. P. (2001). Giving voice to the lifeworld. More humane, more effective medical care? A qualitative study of doctor–patient communication in general practice. *Social Science & Medicine, 53*(4), 487–505. https://doi.org/10.1016/S0277-9536(00)00351-8

Ben-Sira, Z. (1976). The function of the professional's affective behavior in client satisfaction: A revised approach to social interaction theory. *Journal of Health and Social Behavior, 17*(1), 3–11. https://doi.org/10.2307/2136462

Ben-Sira, Z. (1980). Affective and instrumental components in the physician-patient relationship: An additional dimension of interaction theory. *Journal of Health and Social Behavior, 21*(2), 170–180. https://doi.org/10.2307/2136736

Ben-Sira, Z. (1982). Lay evaluation of medical treatment and competence development of a model of the function of the physician's affective behavior. *Social Science & Medicine, 16*(9), 1013–1019. https://doi.org/10.1016/0277-9536(82)90370-7

Burgoon, J. K., & Hale, J. L. (1984). The fundamental topoi of relational communication. *Communication Monographs, 51*(3), 193–214. https://doi.org/10.1080/03637758409390195

Burgoon, J. K., & Hale, J. L. (1987). Validation and measurement of the fundamental themes of relational communication. *Communication Monographs, 54*(1), 19–41. https://doi.org/10.1080/03637758709390214

Burgoon, J. K., & Le Poire, B. A. (1999). Nonverbal cues and interpersonal judgments: Participant and observer perceptions of intimacy, dominance, composure, and formality. *Communications Monographs, 66*(2), 105–124. https://doi.org/10.1080/03637759909376467

Burgoon, J. K., Pfau, M., Parrott, R., Birk, T., Coker, R., & Burgoon, M. (1987). Relational communication, satisfaction, compliance-gaining strategies, and compliance in communication between physicians and patients. *Communication Monographs, 54*(3), 307–324. https://doi.org/10.1080/03637758709390235

Cong, Y. (2004). Doctor-family-patient relationship: The Chinese paradigm of informed consent. *The Journal of Medicine & Philosophy, 29*(2), 149–178. https://doi.org/10.1076/jmep.29.2.149.31506

Conlee, C. J., Olvera, J., & Vagim, N. N. (1993). The relationships among physician nonverbal immediacy and measures of patient satisfaction with physician care. *Communication Reports, 6*(1), 25–33. https://doi.org/10.1080/08934219309367558

Cousin, G., Mast, M. S., Roter, D. L., & Hall, J. A. (2012). Concordance between physician communication style and patient attitudes predicts patient satisfaction. *Patient Education & Counseling, 87*(2), 193–197. https://doi.org/10.1016/j.pec.2011.08.004

Cvengros, J. A., Christensen, A. J., Hillis, S. L., & Rosenthal, G. E. (2007). Patient and physician attitudes in the health care context: Attitudinal symmetry predicts patient satisfaction and adherence. *Annals of Behavioral Medicine, 33*(3), 262–268. https://doi.org/10.1007/BF02879908

Ellis, R. J. B., Carmon, A. F., & Pike, C. (2016). A review of immediacy and implications for provider–patient relationships to support medication management. *Patient Preference and Adherence, 10*, 9–18. https://doi.org/10.2147/PPA.S95163

Epstein, R. M., & Street, R. L. (2007). *Patient-centered communication in cancer care: promoting healing and reducing suffering.* Bethesda, MD: National Cancer Institute.

Finkelstein, A., Carmel, S., & Bachner, Y. G. (2017). Physicians' communication styles as correlates of elderly cancer patients' satisfaction with their doctors. *European Journal of Cancer Care, 26*(1), e12399. https://doi.org/10.1111/ecc.12399

Greene, M. G., & Adelman, R. (2001). Building the physician-older patient relationship. In M. L. Hummert & J. F. Nussbaum (Eds.), *Aging, communication, and health: Linking research and practice for successful aging* (pp. 101–120). Mahwah, NJ: Lawrence Erlbaum Associates.

Greene, M. G., Adelman, R. D., Friedmann, E., & Charon, R. (1994). Older patient satisfaction with communication during an initial medical encounter. *Social Science & Medicine, 38*(9), 1279–1288. https://doi.org/10.1016/0277-9536(94)90191-0

Hall, J. A., Roter, D. L., & Rand, C. S. (1981). Communication of affect between patient and physician. *Journal of Health and Social Behavior, 22*(1), 18–30. https://doi.org/10.2307/2136365

Henry, S. G., Fuhrel-Forbis, A., Rogers, M. A. M., & Eggly, S. (2012). Association between nonverbal communication during clinical interactions and outcomes: A systematic review and meta-analysis. *Patient Education and Counseling, 86*(3), 297–315. https://doi.org/10.1016/j.pec.2011.07.006

Hesse, C., & Rauscher, E. A. (2018). The relationships between doctor–patient affectionate communication and patient perceptions and outcomes. *Health Communication, 34*(8), 881–891. https://doi.org/10.1080/10410236.2018.1439269

Hong, H., & Oh, H. J. (2019). The effects of patient-centered communication: Exploring the mediating role of trust in healthcare providers. *Health Communication, 35*(4), 502–511. https://doi.org/10.1080/10410236.2019.1570427

Inui, T. S., Carter, W. B., Kukull, W. A., & Haign, V. H. (1982). Outcome-based doctor–patient interaction analysis I: Comparison of techniques. *Medical Care, 20*(6), 535–549. https://doi.org/10.1097/00005650-198206000-00001

Ishikawa, H., Takayama, T., Yamazaki, Y., Seki, Y., & Katsumata, N. (2002). Physician-patient communication and patient satisfaction in Japanese cancer consultations. *Social Science & Medicine, 55*(2), 301–311. https://doi.org/10.1016/S0277-9536(01)00173-3

Jahng, K. H., Martin, L. R., Golin, C. E., & DiMatteo, M. R. (2005). Preferences for medical collaboration: patient–physician congruence and patient outcomes. *Patient Education and Counseling, 57*(3), 308–314. https://doi.org/10.1016/j.pec.2004.08.006

Kim, S. S., Kaplowitz, S., & Johnston, M. V. (2004). The effects of physician empathy on patient satisfaction and compliance. *Evaluation & The Health Professions, 27*(3), 237–251. https://doi.org/10.1177%2F0163278704267037

Levenstein, J. H., McCracken, E. C., McWhinney, I. R., Stewart, M. A., & Brown, J. B. (1986). The patient-centred clinical method. 1. A model for the doctor–patient interaction in family medicine. *Family Practice, 3*(1), 24–30. https://doi.org/10.1093/fampra/3.1.24

Mehrabian, A. (1969). Some referents and measures of nonverbal behavior. *Behavior Research Method and Instruction, 1*(6), 203–207. https://doi.org/10.3758/BF03208096

Neuman, W. L. (2011). *Social research methods: Qualitative and quantitative approaches.* Boston: Pearson Education.

Penn, C., & Watermeyer, J. (2012). When asides become central: Small talk and big talk in interpreted health interactions. *Patient Education and Counseling, 88*(3), 391–398. https://doi.org/10.1016/j.pec.2012.06.016

Pun, J. K. H., Chan, E. A., Wang, S., & Slade, D. (2018). Health professional-patient communication practices in East Asia: An integrative review of an emerging field of research and practice in Hong Kong, South Korea, Japan, Taiwan, and Mainland China. *Patient Education & Counseling, 101*(7), 1193–1206. https://doi.org/10.1016/j.pec.2018.01.018

Richmond, V. P., Smith, R. S. Jr., Heisel, A. D., & McCroskey, J. C. (2001). Nonverbal immediacy in the physician/patient relationship. *Communication Research Reports, 18*(3), 211–216. https://doi.org/10.1080/08824090109384800

Sherrill, W. W., Lawson, K. N., & Bednar, H. S. (2020). The act of listening well: Improving communication skills through bibliotherapy. *Health Communication, 35*(14), 1837–1840. https://doi.org/10.1080/10410236.2019.1663584

Stewart, M. (2001). Towards a global definition of patient centered care: The patient should be the judge of patient centered care. *BMJ, 322,* 444–445. https://doi.org/10.1136/bmj.322.7284.444

Tu, J., Kang, G., Zhong, J., & Cheng, Y. (2019). Outpatient communication patterns in a cancer hospital in China: A qualitative study of doctor–patient encounters. *Health Expectations, 22*(3), 594–603. https://doi.org/10.1111/hex.12890

Venetis, M. K., Robbinson, J. D., Turkiewicz, K. L., & Allen, M. (2009). An evidence base for patient-centered cancer care: A meta-analysis of studies of observed communication between cancer specialists and their patients. *Patient Education and Counseling, 77*(3), 379–383. https://doi.org/10.1016/j.pec.2009.09.015

Wang, Q. (2010). *Doctor–patient communication and patient satisfaction: A crosscultural comparative study between China and the US* (Publication No. 3444876) [Doctoral dissertation, Purdue University]. ProQuest Dissertations and Theses Database.

Wanzer, M. B., Booth-Butterfield, M., & Gruber, K. (2004). Perceptions of health care providers' communication: Relationships between patient-centered communication and satisfaction. *Health Communication, 16*(3), 363–384. https://doi.org/10.1207/S15327027HC1603_6

Watson, B. M., & Gallois, C. (1999). Communication accommodation between patients and health professionals: Themes and strategies in satisfying and unsatisfying encounters. *International Journal of Applied Linguistics, 9*(2), 167–180. https://doi.org/10.1111/j.1473-4192.1999.tb00170.x

Wu, Q. L., & Tang, L. (2021). What satisfies parents of pediatric patients in China: A grounded theory building analysis of online physician reviews. *Health Communication*, https://doi.org/10.1080/10410236.2021.1888437

Zimmerman, M. (1993). *A comparison of nonverbally communicated immediacy behaviors in medical interviews of Latino and non-Latino white physicians and patients* (Publication No. 9324522) [Doctoral dissertation, University of San Francisco]. ProQuest Dissertations Publishing.

5 'Come and see me later with your diagnostic test results'

5.1 Introduction

It is widely acknowledged that information on diagnostic testing (e.g., x-rays, blood tests, and imaging) is central to various medical tasks including, but not limited to, information collection, diagnosis, and treatment. It is a common practice for a patient who goes to the doctor's office and presents symptoms to be requested by their doctor to undergo certain diagnostic tests. These tests are considered the most potent tools to confirm or exclude suspected diseases and avoid unnecessary treatment (Goldman et al., 2013). Yet in spite of its importance, diagnostic testing as one of the major activities in medical encounters has been largely underresearched.

Much of the earlier research has considered diagnostic testing a type of treatment decision-making (see Robinson, 2003 in his footnotes) rather than an activity of its own. For example, Pilnick (2008) examined the topicalization of choice (i.e., accepting or declining antenatal screening) in prescreening consultations in the United Kingdom. Rather than focusing on the interactional organization of antenatal screening, the analysis was mainly concerned with the achievement of a decision (see also Pilnick & Zayts, 2016). Similarly, Sterie et al.'s (in press) study on patients' preferences about cardiopulmonary resuscitation addressed diagnostic testing as collaborative treatment-relevant action.

Toerien et al.'s (2020) study on test ordering is the most relevant work to the present study. Using CA, they focused on participants' orientation toward test ordering as a normative activity in first neurology outpatient encounters in the UK. Their major finding is the status of test ordering as an additional activity rather than being part of the treatment decision-making activity in first neurology consultations. Their analysis demonstrated a dual orientation of the test-ordering activity: it can 'simultaneously halt immediate progress toward accomplishing the overarching project and offer hope of future evidence on which to base effective treatment' (Toerien et al., 2000, p. 422).

Despite the importance of diagnostic testing, the overuse or overreliance on medical technology might disrupt doctor–patient interaction and weaken patient care (Lu, 2016). As Iida and Nishigori (2016) noted, the overuse of diagnostic

DOI: 10.4324/9781003161929-5

testing has resulted in the infrequent use of traditional physical examinations such as touching, which displays doctors' empathy, care, and concern about the patient (Kelly et al., 2020). In that sense, diagnostic testing prohibits both interpersonal and physical proximity. Studies have reported an association between fewer diagnostic tests and perceived patient-centeredness (Bertakis et al., 1999; Orom et al., 2018; Stewart et al., 2000). While this scholarship suggests a negative association between diagnostic testing and patient-centeredness, less is known about how diagnostic testing disrupts doctor–patient interactions. Drawing on the findings from the RIAS study (Chapter 3) and the survey results (Chapter 4), this chapter provides a detailed microanalysis of diagnostic testing recommendations in WM visits. In this chapter, I focus on the sequential organization of doctors' diagnostic testing recommendations and the actions such recommendations accomplish in both the here-and-now interaction and the overall medical consultation.

5.2 After patient problem presentation

In his hugely influential study on doctor–patient consultations in acute primary care, Robinson (2003) summed up the core activities related to solving patients' new problems: establishing the reason for the current visit, gathering information through questions and physical examination, delivering a diagnosis, and recommending treatment options. Heritage and Robinson (2006a) further clarified three types of problems: routine acute problems, a recurrent problem similar to a non-routine condition, and unknown problems. While the concept of *problem presentation* was affiliated more with acute consultations and much less with routine consultations, I argue that new problem presentation is not exclusive to acute care encounters, particularly in the care of older patients. Although routine encounters in chronic care provide healthcare service for persistent and long-lasting conditions, these conditions might have some *newness* – either improving or worsening – that distinguishes the problem from the one diagnosed earlier. This might explain the reason that doctors regularly manage diagnostic tests to monitor the patient's condition, particularly in the care of older patients who usually have multiple chronic conditions. In addition, new problem presentations might also occur in routine consultations. For these considerations, the term *problem presentation* is borrowed when analyzing the sequential positions of diagnostic test recommendations.

In the data, doctors usually recommended diagnostic testing after the patient presents their problems. Notably, this activity occurred even before the doctor inquired about the patient's medical history. While Heritage and Clayman (2010) argued that the problem presentation is normally ended up by the doctor's history-taking questions (e.g., questions regarding the duration and details of the pain), in the present WM corpus, there are instances when problem presentation is ended up by a test recommendation. In Extract 1, the patient has some irritable bowel problems. The previous year, she had had surgery for bowel obstruction.

(1) Stool analysis

```
01 D: ai  zenme bu  hao
      hey what  not good
      Hey, what's wrong?

02 P: yisheng wo zuijin   nage Dabian ou  nage dabian
      doctor  I  recently that stools PRT that stools
      Doctor, I recently had that, my Stools, the stools

03    da chulai  yibian   shi  ruan de
      pass out   one side is   soft PRT
      when the stools pass out, one side is soft,

04    yibian   shi  yikeke  de
      one side is   lumps   PRT
      the other side looks like some little lumps.

05    nage aizheng shi bushi (.) ye  shi yikeke        de  a?
      that cancer  is  not      also is  little lumps PRT PRT
      Are these little lumps (.) also a symptom of cancer or not?

06 D: zuo ge  huayan          ou
      do  a   stool analysis PRT
      Take a stool analysis.

07 P: huayan          a?
      stool analysis PRT
      Stool analysis?

08 D: ai
      yep
      Yep.

09 P: nage zhiqian chou le    ge xue
      that earlier take PRT   a blood test
      I had taken a blood test earlier.

10 D: en (.) zai            zuo  ge  huayan         ou
      mmm    additionally do a    stool analysis PRT
      Mmm (.) take a stool analysis additionally.

11 P: ou
      PRT ((indicating agreement))
      Ou.

12 D: qu   liu  ge dabian ou
      go leave a stools PRT
      Leave some stool samples.

13 P: ou
      PRT
      Ou.

14 (0.5) ((the doctor prints the test requisition form))

15 P: jintian zaochen zhege erduo haoxiang qi   a (.)
      today   morning this  ear    seems    air PRT
      This morning, my ears seem like, the air (.)
```

16   shi bushi erduo you   maobing a?
      is not   ears have problem PRT
      Is there something wrong with my ears?

The interview opens with the doctor's general inquiry (Heritage & Robinson, 2006b), making relevant the patient's new-concern presentation (Robinson, 2006). The doctor's question is hearable as having a negative import with the use of *buhao* ('not good'), displaying a problem orientation toward the incipient action. In response to the doctor's new-concern question format, the patient first establishes the reason for the visit by offering a description of her primary symptoms at lines 2 to 4. At first, the patient projects but delays her symptom presentation (her answer with *nage*, line 2), suggesting her difficulty in managing her response. The symptom presentation is then followed immediately with a *candidate diagnosis* (Stivers, 2002), which displays the patient's diagnostic inference of her situation. The two distinct practices (i.e., symptoms-only description and candidate diagnosis) in the patient's turn present her problem with different levels of detail and provide a good account of her diagnostic inference (that the patient had some symptoms similar to a cancer-indicative symptom). Therefore, the patient's problem presentation involves what Schegloff (2000) termed *granularity*: the first part of the turn constitutes a *symptom-only* presentation, whereas the second part constitutes a *candidate diagnosis* (Stivers, 2002). The formulation of the candidate diagnosis in a question format accomplishes two tasks: (1) it mitigates or downgrades the patient's certainty of the diagnostic inference embedded in the candidate diagnosis; and (2) it announces completion of the problem presentation (Robinson & Heritage, 2005) and a transition of activities (Robinson & Stivers, 2001) between *problem presentation* and *diagnosis* by inviting confirmation or disagreement. In other words, the patient might orient themselves toward a diagnosis as the doctor's task in the here-and-now interaction and an area that falls within the doctor's authority (Heritage, 2021; Peräkyla, 2006).

The doctor's recommendation of a stool analysis in the responsive turn (line 6) suggests that the doctor might be oriented to problem presentation as an action that makes diagnostic testing relevant. Although the doctor's test recommendation seems to be misaligned with the patient's diagnosis orientation, it is the stepping-stone for an accurate diagnosis. Studies have indicated the effectiveness of a stool analysis in detecting colorectal cancer (Davies et al., 2005). In that sense, the test recommendation serves a 'both-and' function: it is both a displacement of a diagnosis in the here-and-now interaction and a diagnosis-oriented future action (see Toerien et al., 2020).

The doctor's test recommendations (lines 6, 10, and 12) demonstrate a downward progression of force. In line 6, the formulation of the recommendation in an imperative form displays the doctor's authority and preempts a rejection. Yet, this orientation fails to be immediately aligned by the patient: by offering information on her earlier blood test (line 9), the patient possibly proposes an alternative to the stool analysis. In that sense, acceptance of the test recommendation is delayed, if not rejected. However, the patient's proposal is not accepted by the doctor. Here, the doctor's turn (line 10) accomplishes a couple of interactional tasks simultaneously. First, the neutral, minimal acknowledgment (umm) displays the doctor's attentiveness to the patient. Second, the repetition of the test recommendation strengthens the importance of the recommended test, with the final particle serving as a warning reminder in spoken Chinese (Chao, 2011). Third, the recommendation being reformulated as an action additional to what the patient has proposed mitigates the force of the recommendation by agreeing upon the patient's proposal (blood test) as valuable but not sufficient, making patient acceptance relevant (line 11). Upon the achievement of patient acceptance, the doctor pursues further repetition of the recommendation (line 12) but formulates it in a different manner. The request for the patient to leave some stool samples explains the test procedure and places the stools rather than the patient as the object of the test. The patient again produces *ou*, which registers and minimally accepts the doctor's recommendation and orients to a possible completion of the current symptom (Robinson & Heritage, 2005). In the silence at line 14, the doctor prints the test order form. Together, the patient's assumption of the complete presentation and the absence of the doctor's verbal actions (e.g., question-asking) provide an opportunity for the patient to present her second symptom (lines 15–16).

A similar case is shown in Extract 2. The patient talks with the doctor in the local dialect while the doctor speaks Mandarin, which is reflected in the transcripts. In the extract, in response to the patient's problem presentation (lines 3–5), the doctor agrees with the patient's candidate diagnosis and then recommends a test (line 8).

```
(2) Long-lasting gastritis
01  P: yisheng AI:you
        doctor   PRT
        Doctor, AI:you.

02  D: ni zenme le    a?
        you what PRT PRT
        What's wrong?

03  P: dagai  lao weibing  You    fazuo    d'lei
        Likely old gastritis again attack    PRT
        It's likely the long-lasting gastritis attack Again.

04     YOU    fan   le(.)  zhejitian  teng de  yaoming
        again attack PRT    these days pain PRT kill me
        It attacks me AGAIN (.) these days. It's so painful
        that it almost kills me.

05     ai:you tong a   tong si  d'lei
        PRT    pain PRT pain die PRT
        Ai:you it's so painful.
```

```
06  D: AI::you man     lihai    de   me
         PRT      very  serious PRT PRT
         AI:you it's very serious.
07  P: shi d'lou
         yes PRT
         Yes.
08  D: ni kan   ni  ZUIhao ne  zuo yige weijing
         you see you better PRT take a    gastroscopy
         Look, you'd BEtter take a gastroscopy
09       cha          yixia
         investigate PRT
         for investigation
10  P: ou   haode
         PRT okay
         Ou okay.
11  D: zhezhong   lao weibing haishi   yao
         this kind old gastritis should need
         For such long-lasting gastritis you should,
12       yinggai yao  dingqi    fucha de  xiang ni
         should  need regular review PRT like  you
         you should take regular reviews
11  P: xianzai jiu  qu  a?
         Now      just go PRT
         Shall I go there now?
12  (0.4) ((The doctor types information onto the screen))
13  D: ni zhege you   jitian    le  a?
         you this have some days PRT PRT
         How long is the symptom?
```

This consultation starts with the patient's opening sequence, which is hearable having a negative import with the use of a strongly intonated interjection *AI:you* (Wu, 2016), displaying a problematic orientation toward what comes next. The doctor aligns with the patient's problematic orientation and invites the patient to build his concerns with an open-ended question (line 1). In response to the problem solicitation (line 2), the patient offers a candidate diagnosis (line 3) and then describes his symptoms as evidence for the diagnostic conclusion (line 4). The patient offers as his reason for the visit, the inference that he had a chronic routine concern (Robinson, 2006) via the expression of *You* ('again'), displaying his knowledge about the condition. The patient continues his symptom presentation with an *aiyou*-prefixed turn (line 5), showing his feelings and indicating the seriousness of his situation. The doctor's *aiyou*-prefixed response (1) aligns with the patient's problem orientation, (2) offers an initial assessment of the patient's situation, (3) agrees with the patient's candidate diagnosis, and (4) builds rapport. The accomplishment of these activities in the doctor's responsive turn at line 6 makes a case for her diagnostic test recommendation (lines 8–9), which is immediately accepted by the patient without hesitation (line 10). Thus, both participants demonstrate an orientation toward diagnostic testing as the relevant activity to understanding the patient's condition. This mutual orientation persists to line 11 where the patient indicates compliance with the doctor's test recommendation.

In recommending a test after the patient's problem presentation, the doctor communicates an orientation to the patient's problem as being in need of scientific evidence for diagnosis. This can be seen again in Extract 3. The doctor recommends the patient stay in the hospital and undergo a physical check-up. While patient acceptance is not achieved, the doctor pursues further her recommendation and indicates the importance of a check-up.

```
(3) Dizziness
01 P: yisheng
       doctor
       Doctor.

02 D: en    zenme?
       mmm what's up
       Mmm what's up?

03 P: wo jiushi zongshi juede
       I  just   always  feel
       I just always felt

04 D: en
       mmm
       Mmm.

05 P: wo zhege tou   a jiushi meitian  dou shi
       I  this  head PRT just  everyday all is
       My head just, everyday it is

06     yun (.) yun   huhu de   ganjue tsk
       dizzy   dizzy PRT   PRT feel    tsk
       I felt dizzy, dizzy tsk.

07 D: ni    zong shi zheyang
       you always is  this
       You're always like this.

08     yao wo shuo ni   jiu jinkuai zhuyuan
       If  I  say  you just asap hospitalization
       I would say that you should stay in the hospital asap,

09     zuo ge tijian  chedi      cha    yixia
       take a checkup thorough   check  PRT
       and take a checkup for a thorough investigation.

10 P: wo meinian      dou tijian  de   a
       I  every year  all check-up PRT PRT
       I take a regular check-up every year.

11 D: ni  nage   shequ      tijian
       you that community   check-up
       That one was community-based.
```

```
12  P: wo jiushi [nage
       I    just that
       I'm just [that

13  D:         [zhu    buzhu?
                Stay not
               [Stay or not?

14  P: a?
       ah
       Ah?

15  D: yao buyao zhu?
       Will not   stay
       Will you stay in the hospital or not?

16     zhu   wo jiu gei ni   anpai   le
       stay I will   to you arrange PRT
       If yes, I am gonna arrange that for you.

17  P: wo dei  kaolv    yixia
       I   need consider PRT
       I need to think about it.

18  (0.2)

19     wo ne shuimian ye  bu   hao
       I  PRT sleep   also not  good
       My sleep is not good as well.
```

After the patient registers her presence (line 1), the doctor offers the patient the legitimate right to tell her story via an open question (line 2). The patient gives her primary symptom (lines 3-6), displaying an orientation toward the symptom as the reason for the visit. In response to the patient's telling of her symptom, which is hearable as having some negative import, the doctor aligns with the patient's problem orientation, builds emotional rapport, and displays her knowledge about the patient's condition (line 7). Immediately after that, she adds two other turn-constructional units (TCUs) (Sacks et al., 1974), recommending diagnostic testing as the relevant and immediate ('asap') action that the patient should do next (lines 8–9). Notably, while two actions are suggested in the doctor's test recommendation (hospitalization and physical check-up), they are considered closely related: a thorough investigation of the patient's health is framed as the purpose of hospitalization. Here, the doctor displays an orientation toward the patient's problem as in need of a detailed investigation. This orientation is more pronounced in her next turn (line 11) where patient acceptance is not achieved (line 10), and the doctor indicates a difference between the recommended test and the community test that the patient has undergone regularly. In this sense, the doctor pursues further her prior test recommendation. Interestingly, where the doctor's pursuit of the test recommendation is not attended to by the patient (line 12), the doctor asks a straightforward A-not-A type of question (Gasde, 2004), making relevant patient acceptance or declination. Note here that the doctor's A-not-A type of question is an interruption: it starts at a point that is not a legitimate transition relevant place – a projectable completion point of a TCU (see Hutchby, 2008; Schegloff, 2001). While the patient might have failed to catch the doctor's question and requested repetition (line 14), the doctor first repeats the A-not-A question (line 15) and then offers a direction on a future arrangement (line 16). Here, we can see a strengthening force of the doctor's question: while the first A-not-A question is a request for confirmation, the second A-not-A question that followed with an arrangement for future activities is stronger and more rushed (in terms of immediacy). Such immediacy in action aligns with the doctor's earlier action at line 8, where she suggests the patient stay in the hospital as soon as possible. Again, the patient declines the doctor's test recommendation, albeit in a mitigated manner (line 16). By borrowing some time for consideration, the patient politely declines the doctor's recommendation in the here-and-now interaction and indicates a possible future activity. After a short silence (line 18), the patient starts her second problem presentation.

I have provided three extracts where the doctor recommends a test after the patient's problem presentation. The test recommendation takes the place of history-taking. In the first two extracts, the patient accepts the doctor's recommendation, suggesting a mutual orientation toward the relevance of diagnostic testing to the patient's problem. In the third extract, patient acceptance is not obtained. Extract 3 also differs from the first two extracts in how the patient presents their problem: in Extract 3, the patient gives a symptom-only presentation with no 'priori' knowledge of her situation, whereas the patient in the first two extracts seems to have a better understanding of their conditions by indicating their diagnostic inferences (Stivers, 2002). In that sense, while the patient in the first two extracts display their diagnosis orientation, the patient in Extract 3 does not. This might explain the patient's declination of the doctor's test recommendation.

5.3 After the patient's orientation toward the relevance of diagnostic testing

Unlike patients in acute care, patients with chronic conditions usually have previous diagnostic test experiences related to their conditions. For diseases such as gastritis and cancer, regular diagnostic tests are required to monitor patients' condition. In several observations, the patient display their orientation toward the relevance of diagnostic testing for understanding their condition and monitoring the progress. Consider Extracts 4–6. In Extract 4, the patient has colorectal polyps removed one year earlier.

```
(4) Colorectal polyps
01  D: jintian zenme le?
        today    what  PRT
        Why you're here today?
02  P: yisheng a (.) wo gen ni  shuo ou
        doctor PRT    I  to you say   PRT
        Doctor (.) let me tell you.
```

```
03      wo me   shangci   zuo  le   ge changing
        I  PRT last time take PRT   a colonoscopy
        Last time, I took a colonoscopy,
04      name zai zheli huayan    ou
        then at   here  lab test PRT
        then the lab test here.
05  D:  en
        mmm
        Mmm.
06  P:  wo nage zhichangxirou      me jiu shi
        I  that colorectal polyps  PRT just is
        I was told that I had colorectal polyps
07  D:  shenme Shihou zuo  de     changing?
        what   time   take PRT colonoscopy
        When did you take the colonoscopy?
08  P:  shenme shihou a?
        what   time   PRT
        When?
09  D:  ai (.) ni shangci   zuo   Dagai        shi shenme shihou?
        yep    you last time take approximately is  what   time
        Yep (.) approximately when did you take it last time?
10  P:  na    you yi< yinian    duo le   lei
        that  have one one year more PRT PRT
        That's one < more than one year.
11  D:  yinian    duo le    a?
        one year more PRT PRT
        More than one year?
12  P:  ai
        yep
        Yep.
13  D:  na    zai  zuo   yige fucha  yixia haoba?
        then again take  one  review PRT   okay
        Then take one more again, okay?
14  P:  wo xiang zuo  wutong    de
        I  want  take painless PRT
        I want to take a painless one.
15      shangci   zuo de wo TONG a   tong si  le
        last time take PRT I  pain PRT pain die PRT
        Last time, it was too painful.
```

The doctor's opening elicitation of the patient's agenda invokes an extensive presentation of the patient's concern (lines 2–6). The patient's telling of his symptoms is formulated to show his orientation toward the relevance of diagnostic testing for understanding his condition and diagnosis. By naming the test of a colonoscopy (line 3), the patient indicates his knowledge about the function of the test. In response to the patient's telling of his story, the doctor asks the patient for further information about his earlier test (line 7), displaying an alignment with the patient's orientation. While the patient seems to have difficulty preparing his answer (line 8), the doctor reformulates her question by suggesting an approximation in the patient's answer (line 9). After patient information-giving (lines 10–12), the doctor advises the patient to take the test again for an update (line 13). The patient's request for a painless test indicates his acceptance of the doctor's recommendation. Extract 5 shows a similar sequence.

```
(5) Swollen stomach
01 D: ni zenme bu hao?
      you what not good
      What's wrong?
02 P: wo zhege Wei (.)     zhang
      I    this stomach    swell
      My Stomach swells.
03    wo zhiqian   zuo  guo  weijing       de
      I  previous take have gastroscopy PRT
      I had taken the gastroscopy before.
04 D: ni  weijing      baogao ne?
      you gastroscopy report PRT?
      Where's your gastroscopy report?
05 P: weijing      ni zheli cha    de  chu de
      gastroscopy you here check PRT out PRT
      You can check that on your screen.
06    weijing      baogao bu zhidao zai        bu    zai
      gastroscopy report no know    available not available
      Not sure if the report can be found or not.
07 D: >na    chulai    na     chulai<
       take outside take outside
      >Take it out, take it out.<
08    ni  na fangbian     yidian
      you take convenient a little
      It would be more convenient if you could show me the report.
09 (0.7)
10 D: ni zhege liang nian   le
      you this two    years PRT
      It was taken two years ago.
11 P: en
      mmm
      Mmm.
12 D: ni  yaoburan    zai  zuo  yige ba
      you how about again take one  PRT
      How about you take another gastroscopy?
13 P: zai     zuo yige a?
      again take one PRT?
      Take another gastroscopy?
```

```
14  D: ai: wo xianzai jiu  gei ni   yuyue (.) haoba
       yep I   now      just for you book    okay
       Ye:p I can book that for you now (.) okay?
```

In response to the doctor's general inquiry inviting patient presentation, the patient first produces a symptom-only presentation (line 1). Then the patient adds in her turn a second TCU (line 3), which displays her orientation toward the relevance of a gastroscopy to her condition. The doctor aligns with the patient's orientation by asking the patient about the test report. 'Where's your gastroscopy report?' It is evident that the doctor would like to read the report for a better understanding of the patient's condition. Thus far, the doctor and the patient display a mutual orientation toward the gastroscopy report as an important source of information. In the next few exchanges (lines 5–8), the doctor and the patient try to find the earlier test report.

The doctor's comment on the earlier test date (line 10) indicates her understanding of the information reported on the test outcome as out of date and insufficient, making a case for her test recommendation (line 12). Although the recommendation on taking another gastroscopy is hearable to seek patient opinions, it is designed for acceptance (see Schegloff, 2007 for the concept of *preference*). The doctor's preference for patient acceptance is more pronounced at line 14, where she proposes an immediate action of scheduling the test.

Extract 6 is different from the previous two extracts. In Extract 6, the patient makes an explicit request for a diagnostic test, which, however, is considered by the doctor as not suitable. In return, the doctor recommends another test, which the patient accepts.

```
(6) H. pylori breath tests or gastroscopy
01  P: yisheng wo lai  zuo yige nage nage
       doctor  I   come take a    that that
       Doctor, I came here to take the the
02     youmenluoxuanganjun
       H. pylori
       H. pylori.
03  D: youmenluoxuanganjun a?
       helicobacter pylori PRT?
       H. pylori?
04  P: ai
       yep
       Yep.
05  D: ni zenme?
       you what
       What's wrong with you?
06  P: wo qunian    cha     chulai shuo milan   me
       I   last year examine outcome say erosive PRT
       I was diagnosed with erosive gastritis last year.
```

```
07      name wo xiang yinian   le  wo   pa    you   jun
        so   I think one year PRT I   afraid have bacteria
        So I think it's been a year.
        I'm worried about the H. pylori.

08      bushi shuo nage jun       zhi   ai    me
        don't say  that bacteria lead to cancer PRT
        Isn't that bacteria a cause of cancer?

09 D:   aizheng xingcheng you henduo yinsu   de
        cancer  form       have a lot factor PRT
        Cancer is caused by several factors.

10      ni   yaome      zuo ge weijing?
        you how about take a gastroscopy
        How about taking the gastroscopy?

11      gei ni   ba youmenluoxuanganjun yiqi    jiancha jinqu
        for you PRT H. pylori            together examine include
        We can include the H. pylori test as well.

12 P:   yiqi       a?
        together PRT
        All in one?

13 D:   ai
        yep
        Yep.

14 P:   ye   keyi ou
        also can  PRT
        That's okay.
```

The patient's request for an H. pylori test at the beginning of the consultation displays her orientation toward diagnostic testing as being the reason for her visit. However, the doctor's agreement is not immediately produced. Instead, the doctor seeks the reason for the patient's request (line 5), providing another opportunity for the patient to present her problems. As a response to the doctor's question, the patient first provides information on her earlier diagnosis (line 6). Immediately after that, in the first TCU of her line at 7, she offers temporal information about her condition, indicating a need for a review. Then, in the second TCU, she expresses her primary concern: 'I am worried about the H. pylori', indicating her orientation toward a diagnostic test. The patient's assertion of the causality between H. pylori and cancer (line 8) explains her concern and emphasizes her orientation toward the relevance of the H. pylori test to identify or rule out cancer.

As a response to the patient's request, the doctor first corrects the patient's understanding of cancer (line 9), displaying a problem orientation toward the patient's assertion and building a case for her test recommendation (line 10). By indicating the inclusion of a H. pylori test in the recommended alternative test (line 11), the doctor (1) attends to the patient's concern, (2) fulfils her institutional task of test recommendation, and (3) makes patient acceptance relevant (line 14).

5.4 After history-taking questions

The history-taking phase of the interaction is pivotal to medical diagnosis (Stoeckle & Billings 1987). It provides information about the two worlds of the patient: the medical world and the lifeworld (see the concept of *world* in Cole & Bird, 2013). As Boyd and Heritage (2006) stated, the history provides a 'historical context' (p. 152) for the doctor to understand their patients and make a diagnosis. In the data, I found that after the doctor produces the first couple of history-taking questions, a test recommendation is offered, functioning as supportive evidence of the patient's history for diagnosis. Consider Extracts 7–9. In Extract 7, prior to line 1, the patient tells the doctor that he had rectal pain for around a month.

```
(7) Rectal pain
01 D: ni zhege difang teng le  duojiu    le?
       you this place   pain PRT how long PRT
       How long is the pain here?
02 P: yige yue
       one  month
       One month.
03 D: yige yue?
       one month
       One month?
04 P: yige yue    zuoyou ba
       one  month around PRT
       Around one month.
05 D: yiqian teng bu teng de?
       past    pain no pain PRT
       Did you feel painful in the past?
06 P: yiqian ye    teng guo   de
       past    also pain have PRT
       It was painful in the past.
07 D: na    zuizao kaishi shihou teng   duojiu  ne?
       then earliest begin when    pain how long PRT
       How long the pain lasted at the very earliest beginning?
08 P: teng teng duojiu (.) ye    hen   jiu
       pain pain how long   also very long
       How long the pain, pain, it also lasted long.
09 D: ni zheyang gei ni    zuo yige changjing
       you this    for you take one colonoscopy
       Let's take a colonoscopy.
10 P: changjing      a?
       colonoscopy PRT
       Colonoscopy?
```

```
11  D: ai (.) bu paichu    you xirou   ou
        yep     no exclude have polyps PRT
        Yep (.) we cannot exlude the possibility of polyps.

12      zuo ge changjing    jiancha yixia
        take a colonoscopy check    PRT
        Take a colonoscopy to check.

13  P: ou
        PRT
        Ou.
```

As a response to the patient's problem presentation (data not shown), the doctor asks several history-taking questions, using a mixture of closed- and open-ended questions, including questions on the duration of the pain (line 1) and the earlier symptoms (lines 5–7). These questions aimed at collecting information about the patient's condition in more detail, display the doctor's orientation toward the current interaction as history-taking. After understanding the progression of the patient's symptoms, the doctor recommends the patient undergo a colonoscopy (line 9). Unlike previous extracts where the doctor's test recommendation is framed in a mitigated and polite manner by seeking patient acceptance, the test recommendation here is designed in imperatives, preempting patient declination. While acceptance is withheld in the patient's responsive turn (line 10), the doctor explains her test recommendation – to detect or exclude the possibility of polyps. Note that the doctor's explanatory utterance at line 11 could also be understood as her initial diagnosis of the patient's condition, which is yet to be proved by scientific evidence. Immediately after that, in the next TCU of her turn, the doctor tells the patient the purpose of the test, building connections between test recommendation and diagnosis. In so doing, the doctor also displays her orientation toward the patient's condition as being in need of scientific investigation. In response to the doctor's advice, the patient indicates acceptance via the minimum acknowledgment token 'ou' (line 13).

```
(8) Functional gastrointestinal disorder
01  D: dabian hao    bu hao?
        poop   good no good
        Is your poop good or bad?

02  P: dabian haihao
        poop    not bad
        It's not bad.

03      Haiyou   me jiushi youshihou youdian   tong de
        besides PRT just   sometimes a little pain PRT
        In addition, it felt pain sometimes.

04  D: weijing     zuo  guo  ma?
        gasroscopy take have PRT
        Have you taken gastroscopy before?
```

```
05  P:  zuo guo de
        take past PRT
        I took one before.
06  D:  gei wo kankan
        to  me look
        Give it to me.
07  (0.4)
08  P:  weijing      me   yiqian  de  le
        gastroscopy PRT earlier PRT PRT
        It was taken earlier.
09  D:  15 nian zuo de
        15 year take PRT
        It was taken in 2015.
10  P:  ai: HAO      jinian      le
        yep quite many years PRT
        Ye:p QUITE a few years ago.
11  D:  ni    zai zuo  yige ba (.) zhege tai zao    le
        you again take one PRT      this too early PRT
        You take the test again (.) this one was too early.
12  P:  tai zao    le ou?
        too early PRT PRT
        Too early?
13  D:  en
        mmm
        Mmm.
14  P:  ou    na  jiu  zai   zuo yige
        PRT then just again take one
        Ou then I shall take the test again.
15  (0.5)
16  D:  qita  you nali  bu  shufu      ma
        other have where not comfortable PRT
        Anywhere else that you feel uncomfortable?
```

Prior to line 1, the patient tells the doctor that her primary concern is a distended abdomen and hiccup (data not shown). In response to the patient's problem presentation, the doctor produces a yes/no interrogative asking the patient if her bowel movements were normal. Thereafter, the doctor produces a second yes/no interrogative, asking the patient about her past test experience. The successive use of yes/no questions to collect information from the patient displays the doctor's orientation toward the current interaction as history-taking. The doctor's request for the patient's earlier gastroscopy report (line 6) indicates her orientation toward the test report as being indicative of the patient's condition, paving the ground for her subsequent recommendation of retesting.

Upon achieving the mutual orientation between the doctor and the patient toward the outdatedness of the patient's earlier gastroscopy report (lines –10), the doctor suggests the patient take the test again, as evidenced in her second TCU at line 11. The patient agreed with the doctor and accepted the recommendation (line 14). After patient acceptance, the doctor pursued further information collection by eliciting additional concerns of the patient.

In Extracts 7 and 8, a strong orientation toward the recentness of diagnostic testing is displayed by the doctor. Such orientation is made more pronounced in Extract 9, where the doctor indicates her disagreement with the patient showing her the test report that was produced the previous year. Prior to line 1, the patient tells the doctor that she always had nausea.

```
(9)  It was last year
01  D: ni    shangci   weijing      zuo  mei zuo   la?
        you  last time gastroscopy take not take  PRT
        Did you take the gastroscopy or not last time?

02  P: zuo   le  de
        take PRT PRT
        Yes I did.

03  D: shenme shihou zuo   de?
        what   time   take PRT
        When did you take the test?

04  P: e:: qunian
        uhm last year
        Uh::m last year.

05  D: qunian    shenme shihou?
        last year what   time
        What time last year?

06  P: qi- qiyuefen ba
        July July       PRT
        Ju- July.

07  D: qunian    qiyuefen? YI nian  Ban  a?
        last year July     one year half PRT
        Last July? ONE year and Half?

08  P: ai
        yep
        Yep.

09  D: zai    zuo yige
        again take one
        Do it again.

10  P: zhege shi qunian     zuo  de
        this  is  last year take PRT
        This is last year's test report

11  D: ni  QUnian    de  baogao ni XIANzai gei wo
        you last year PRT report you now     to  me
        You show me Now the report that was made LAST year.

12  P: wo xiang wo mei gei ni   kan guo   ma    hehe
        I  think I  not to  you look have PRT   hh-hh
        I'm thinking that I haven't showed you the report heh heh.
```

```
13  D:  yinian     Ban  le  (.)
        one year  half  PRT
        It's one year and Half.
14      weijing      haishi zai   zuo  yige  ba   haoba
        gastroscopy better again take one   PRT  okay
        You'd better take one more again, okay?
15  P:  yaome yao        chi chi hao  bu   hao?
        or    medicine eat eat okay not  okay
        Or just take some medicine okay?
```

The doctor's yes/no interrogative on patient experience of gastroscopy marks the transition (Robinson & Stivers, 2001) from problem presentation to history-taking. The doctor then proceeds with a list of questions seeking information specification regarding when the patient underwent her last gastroscopy (lines 3–7). In so organizing the discussion, the doctor displays her orientation toward the importance of the recentness of diagnostic testing in understanding the patient's condition, making the basis for her test recommendation. After indicating a possible surprise on the outdatedness of the patient's last test report – evidenced by the intonated temporal reference at line 7 – the doctor produces a test recommendation that is hearable as an imperative or directive (line 9). The design of the doctor's test recommendation reflects her orientation toward the patient's condition as being in need of an updated test for diagnosis.

Interesting to note is the doctor's response to the patient's negative results for her earlier test at lines 10–11. The doctor's intonated tone on the contrasted temporal reference ('NOW' and 'LAST year') in her response displays disagreement with the patient and indicates her orientation toward the test report as being not convincing. This orientation persists to her next turn at lines 13–14, where the doctor re-comments on the outdatedness of the patient's earlier report and proposes retaking the test.

In this extract, the doctor twice provides a recommendation on retaking a gastroscopy: lines 9 and 14, with a progression of negotiability and politeness. In line 15, the recommendation is made in imperatives, which is hearable as being directive and less negotiable, making patient compliance relevant. At line 14, possibly as a response to the patient's affiliative laughter (Jefferson et al., 1987), the doctor's second test recommendation is provided, formulated to seek patient agreement (preferred) or disagreement (not preferred) with the articulation of 'okay?'

5.5 'Come and see me later with your diagnostic test results'

In several observations, patient acceptance of the doctor's test recommendation makes relevant a temporary closing of the encounter. The encounter usually resumes after the patient completes the recommended test. Extract 10 is a full episode of the consultation. The patient has multiple chronic conditions, including high amylase levels and high blood pressure. She had undergone an

MRI and CT two years earlier and has since then taken medication. The doctor's diagnostic recommendation is provided on lines 16–17.

(10) Elevated amylase level

```
01  P:  yisheng  wo  jiu  shi  dianfenmei      gao  la
        doctor   I   just am  amylase levels  high PRT
        Doctor, I'm just, my amylase levels are high.

02  D:  en
        mmm
        Mmm.

03  P:  dianfenmei      gao me (.) qunian
        Amylase levels high PRT    last year
        My amylase level is high (.) last year.

04      zuo  le  yici cigongzhen yixian     de     ou
        take PRT once MRI         pancreas  PRT    PRT
        I took an MRI to investigate my pancreas.

05  D:  en
        mmm
        Mmm.

06  P:  name   jinnian    ne    haishi gao
        then   this year  PRT   still  high
        Then, this year, it's still high.

07  (0.5)

08  D:  zhe  shi shenme shihou? 16 nian 12 yue
        this is  what   time    16 year 12 month
        When did you take the test? In Dec. 2016.

09      dianfenmei zonggui    shi pian     gao     yidian
        amylase    after all  is  relatively high  a little
        The amylase level was higher than normal after all.

10  P:  en
        mmm
        Mmm.

11  D:  qunian     jiu     kaishi le  shiba?
        last year already start   PRT right
        It started last year, right?

12  P:  Ai: qunina
        yep last year
        YE:p last year.

13      qunian     yinwei    pian      gao suoyi zuo cigongzhen me
        last year because relatively high so    take MRI       PRT
        Since it was found higher than normal last year,
        I took the MRI.

14  D:  zhege shi CT
        this  is  CT
        This is CT.
```

```
15  P:  haiyou        yige cigongzhen
        in addition one    MRI
        I took MRI as well.

16  D:  ni   zhege qingkuang  mei    sange yue
        you this  condition every three month
        Given your condition, every three months

17      yao  lai  fucha           yi  ci  de
        need come re-examination one time PRT
        you need to take the test again.

18  P:  mei    sangeyue       a?
        every three months PRT
        Every three months?

19  D   en (.)  mei    sangeyue   chou    yici xue (.)
        mmm    every three months collect once blood
        Mmm(.) take a blood test every three months,

20      xianzai jiu   qu chou    yige
        now     just go collect one
        go and take the  blood test now.

21  P:  xianzai jiu   qu  a?
        now     just go PRT
        Go there now?

22  D:  ai  xian qu jiaofei ranhou yilou     chouxue
        yep first go  pay   then   first floor blood test
        Yep first you go to the cashier and then go to the
            first floor for the blood test.

23      chou    hao zai    guolai
        Collect end again    come
        Come to me again after that.

24  P:  ou haode
        PRT okay
        Ou okay.
```

This consultation opens with the patient's extensive problem presentation (lines 1–6), divided into several parts. At first, the patient's problem is presented (line 1) as both a symptom-only description and candidate diagnosis: on the one hand, the elevated amylase level can be a symptom indicating some illnesses. On the other hand, it could also be a diagnosis based on scientific evidence (see lines 3–4). The doctor's articulation of *umm* at line 2 functions as a backchannel, offering the patient the legitimate right to continue his telling. As a response to the doctor's backchannel invitation, the patient continues his telling, making reference to his earlier test results (lines 3–4). Notably, the information on earlier test results, the use of a temporal reference ('last year') marks an activity transition between problem presentation and history-taking. The doctor aligns with the patient's orientation by asking a typical history-taking question: 'when did you take the test?' (line 8). Immediately after that, the doctor adds a second TCU in her turn and produces a self-correction (Schegloff et al., 1977). This mutual alignment invokes a few exchanges on the patient's amylase level and her earlier diagnostic test (lines 11–15).

The doctor's first advice on regularly doing a diagnostic test occurs at lines 16–17. 'Given your condition, every three months you need to retake the test.' At first glance, the advice is formulated in a way that is hearable as health promotion, built on an assessment of the patient's condition. In her next turn (lines 19–20), the doctor reformulates the advice, naming a specific diagnostic test ('blood test') as a regular practice for the patient and requesting the patient take a blood test in the here-and-now interaction. In other words, the doctor's second advice on a blood test (line 19) can be treated as a reification of her first advice. Interestingly, the conversation temporarily closes at line 24 with the patient accepting the doctor's test recommendation.

The same pattern can be seen in Extracts 11 and 12. In Extract 11, the doctor recommends the patient have a blood test. The patient has chronic gastritis. Prior to line 1, the patient tells the doctor that she recently experienced nausea and sweating. She had a cold these days, which aggravated her symptoms.

```
(11) Nausea and sweating
01  D: duzitong          a      zhexie meiyou de   ou?
        abdominal pain PRT    this   no      PRT PRT
        You don't have symptoms such as abdominal pain?
02  P: na    meiyou de
        that no       PRT
        No I don't,
03      jiushi wei        nanshou
        just   stomach uncomfortable
        just the stomach felt uncomfortable.
04      youshihou gan    ye   you  yidian
        sometimes liver also have a little
        Sometimes the liver also felt a little.
05  D: youshihou ganmao ye    hui  you zhezhong
        Sometimes cold    also will have such
        Sometimes cold can also have such
06      wei      chang     de biaoxian de   ou
        stomach intestine PRT symptom PRT PRT
        symptoms reflected on stomach and intestine
07  P: ou: wei         chang     ye   hui
        PRT stomach intestine also will
        Ou: it will also be reflected on the stomach and intestine.
08  D: yaobu      ni   xian yangexue   ba
        what about you first blood test PRT
        What about you take a blood test first
09      [kankan] you meiyou ganran (.) yanzheng     shenme de
        see       have not   infection inflammation such  PRT
        [to see] if you have an infection (.) such like inflammation?
```

```
10  P:  [ou haode]
        PRT okay
        [Ou okay.]
11  D:  chou      hao   xue   hou   guolai
        collect finish blood after come
        After the blood collection come here again,
12      women zai   kan ganmao ou
        we    then see  cold   PRT
           and we deal with the cold
13  P:  haode haode
        okay  okay
        Okay okay.
```

The doctor's closed-ended question at line 1 displays her orientation toward the current interaction as history-taking, seeking to exclude other symptoms of the patient. The question is hearable as preferring a disagreement. The patient aligns with the doctor's orientation by denying the abdominal pain and, immediately in her second TCU, she presents other symptoms (occasional liver disturbance) to help the doctor better understand her condition. In response to the patient's information-giving, the doctor normalizes the patient's condition and provides possible explanations (lines 5–6). While the patient accepts the doctor's explanation, the doctor offers a blood test recommendation (line 8), using a *wh*-question, making patient acceptance relevant. In her next TCU, the doctor provides explanations for her advice, indicating the function of the test. Upon patient acceptance, the doctor makes arrangements for the following activities (lines 11–12) related to the current consultation. The consultation temporarily closes with the patient's acceptance.

Different from Extracts 10 and 11 where the patient came back to the doctor after the test, the patient in Extract 12 left the hospital. Therefore, test recommendation, upon its acceptance, constitutes the last activity of the encounter. In Extract 12, the patient had surgery the previous year to remove rectal polyps and a tumor. Before line 1, the patient tells the doctor that he recently has had a constant urge to pass a stool.

```
(12) Polyps and tumor
01  D:  ou  changjing    jinnian  you meiyou fucha       guo?
        PRT colonoscopy this year have not   retake test have
        Ou did you take the colonoscopy again this year?
02  P:  meiyou
        no
        No.
03  D:  name jianyi  ni  haishi fucha         yixia ou
        then suggest you better re-examination PRT   PRT
        Then I would suggest you take it again.
```

```
04  P:  ye    bu    yiding   °shi [shenme°
        also  not   necessary is   what
        It is not necessarily °[what°
05  D:                            [Dui (.) danshi yinwei    ni    chi
                                   right       but   because you   eat
                                  [Right (.) but because you're having
06      nage zhongliu shuhou         suoyi yao    fucha
        that    tumor post-surgery so     need   re-take test
        the post-surgery medicication, you need to retake the test.
07      changgui ye   yao   meinian    fucha   de
        normally also need  yearly    re-take PRT
        Normally a yearly test re-taking is required.
08  P:  ou (.) changjing jiushi   you    dian      pa
        PRT    colonoscopy just have a little scared
        Ou (.) I'm a little bit scared about colonoscopy.
09  D:  yiban    wutong    de haihao
        usually painless PRT fine
        Usually the painless colonoscopy is fine.
10  P:  ou shenme shihou zuo      a?
        PRT what    time   take PRT
        Ou when do I take the test?
11  D:  yihuier xian  qu fukuan ranhou qu sanlou
        later   first go pay     then   go third floor
        Later you go to the cashier first and then the third floor.
12  P:  zai   huilai     a?
        then come back PRT
        And then come back?
13  D:  ni deng nage baogao  chulai    hou
        you wait that report come out after
        Wait until the report comes out.
14  P:  na   wo zhijie    zou   le    a?
        then I  directly leave PRT
        Then I  would leave after the test,
15      daoshihou zai    guolai?
        by then    again come
        and come here again by then?
16  D:  ai
        yep
        Yep.
17  P:  na   bu yong chi shenme yao       a shenme   de   a?
        then no need eat what    medicine PRT what   PRT PRT
        No need to take medications?
18  D:  deng nage baogao chulai     zai kan ou
        wait that report come out then see PRT
        Wait till the report is ready, and let's see.
```

```
19  P: ou deng baogao
       PRT wait report
       Ou wait for the report.
```

In response to the patient's problem presentation, the doctor asks the patient whether he had undergone colonoscopy this year, displaying an orientation toward the diagnostic test as evidence for understanding the patient's condition. While the patient's response is dispreferred, the doctor advises the patient to repeat the test for regular follow-ups (line 3). The patient's response – 'it is not necessarily [what'] – reflects his understanding of the doctor's test recommendation as having negative import (e.g., suggesting tumor recurrence). By suggesting the possibility of other explanations for his physical symptoms (the constant urge to pass a stool), the patient indicates his declination or disagreement with the doctor's test recommendation. The doctor makes further efforts to persuade the patient: at line 5, she first agrees with the patient's understanding of the existence of other possibilities. Immediately after that, connected with the adversative conjunction 'but', the doctor adds a second TCU, promoting regular diagnostic testing. By building a causative relation between regular diagnostic testing and post-surgery medication through using 'because', the doctor explains to the patient the role of regular diagnostic testing in monitoring patient health. The third TCU (line 7) further strengthens the importance of regular diagnostic testing by normalizing the practice as yearly based. The doctor's further pursuit of recommending a test is first reciprocated with a neutral minimum acknowledgment 'ou' (line 8). The patient's telling of his emotional concerns could be a mitigated declination of the test recommendation. Yet, it is also likely that by indicating his fear about the test, the patient is explaining the reasons for his non-immediate acceptance (line 4) of the doctor's advice about retaking the test. Similarly, the doctor's comment on the painless colonoscopy at line 9 could be either a further pursuit of a test recommendation or an alignment with the patient's emotional concerns.

Note that upon the patient's indication of acceptance (line 10) via the minimum acknowledgment 'ou', the doctor proceeds to arrange for the following activities: payment and a colonoscopy. This arrangement announcement (line 11) functions as a pre-closing (Schegloff & Sacks, 1973), indicating a possible closing of the current encounter. The doctor's closing orientation is made more explicit at line 13: in response to the patient's question regarding the subsequent arrangement, the doctor tells him to visit her at an appointment after the test report was ready. In other words, the doctor indicates a no-further-activity orientation for the current encounter. This orientation is reannounced at line 19 where the doctor suggests no prescription at this stage.

5.6 Summary

In the last two chapters, we see that WM consultations feature frequent talk of diagnostic testing and that such talk may displace history-taking to understand the patient's condition. In the present chapter, we can begin to see how diagnostic testing is recommended in TCM consultations. Put simply, a diagnostic test recommendation occurs in an environment where the doctor perceives a need to either identify or exclude possible diseases, particularly when the symptoms are recurrent. As the name suggests, a test is used for diagnosis. Since the patients for this study are people with chronic conditions, they already know their conditions. In presenting their problems to the doctor, the patient most often provides a candidate diagnosis that could be either a recurrence of a chronic disease or a newly observed symptom of some other unpleasant disease. In such situations, the doctor recommends diagnostic testing to help understand the patient's condition. Alternatively, and in most circumstances, diagnostic testing is suggested as a normal practice for regular medical follow-ups of the patient's past surgery. The advice is offered when the doctor realizes an extended period of time has passed since the patient's last diagnostic test. In such situations, the doctor pursues further health promotion and highlights the importance of regular testing in monitoring the patient's chronic condition. One particular sequential consequence of testing recommendation is that its acceptance makes a temporary closing of the current interaction relevant. Most often, the consultation resumes after the patient completes the test. However, a test recommendation can also make a closure of the encounter relevant (Extract 12) if no other patient issues are to be addressed.

References

Bertakis, K. D., Azari, R., Callahan, E. J., Helms, J., & Robbins, J. A. (1999). The impact of physician practice on medical charges. *The Journal of Family Practice, 48*(1), 31–36.

Boyd, E., & Heritage, J. (2006). Taking the history: Questioning during comprehensive history-taking. In J. Heritage & D. W. Maynard (Eds.), *Communication in medical care: Interaction between primary care physicians and patients* (pp. 151–184). Cambridge: Cambridge University Press. https://doi.org/10.1017/CBO9780511607172.008

Chao, Y. R. (2011). *A grammar of spoken Chinese.* Beijing: The Commercial Press.

Cole, S. A., & Bird, J. (2013). *The medical interview: The three function approach* (3rd ed.). Philadelphia: Elsevier.

Davies, R. J., Miller, R., & Coleman, N. (2005). Colorectal cancer screening: Prospects for molecular stool analysis. *Nature Reviews Cancer, 5*, 199–209. https://doi.org/10.1038/nrc1569

Gasde, H-D. (2004). Yes/no questions and A-not-A questions in Chinese revisited. *Linguistics, 42*(2), 293–326. https://doi.org/10.1515/ling.2004.010

Goldman, D. P., Gupta, C., Vasudeva, E., Trakas, K., Riley, R., Lakdawalla, D., Agus, D., Sood, N., Jena, A. B., & Philipson, T. L. (2013). The value of diagnostic testing in personalized medicine. *Forum for Health Economics and Policy, 16*(2), S97–S99. https://doi.org/10.1515/fhep-2013-0023

Heritage, J. (2021). The expression of authority in US primary care: Offering diagnoses and recommending treatment. In C. Gordon (Ed.), *Approaches to discourse analysis* (pp. 104–122). Washington, DC: Georgetown University Press.

Heritage, J., & Clayman, S. (2010). *Talk in action: Interactions, identities, and institutions.* Oxford: Wiley-Blackwell.

Heritage, J., & Robinson, J. D. (2006a). Accounting for the visit: Giving reasons for seeking medical care. In J. Heritage & D. W. Maynard (Eds.), *Communication in medical care: Interaction between primary care physicians and patients* (pp. 48–85). Cambridge: Cambridge University Press. https://doi.org/10.1017/CBO9780511607172.005

Heritage, J., & Robinson, J. D. (2006b). The structure of patients' presenting concerns: Physicians' opening questions. *Health Communication, 19*(2), 89–102. https://doi.org/10.1207/s15327027hc1902_1

Hutchby, I. (2008). Participants' orientations to interruptions, rudeness and other impolite acts in talk-in-interaction. *Journal of Politeness Research, 4*(2), 221–241. https://doi.org/10.1515/JPLR.2008.011

Iida, J., & Nishigori, H. (2016). Physical examination and the physician–patient relationship: A literature review. *MedEdPublish, 5*(3), 14. https://doi.org/10.15694/mep.2016.000100

Jefferson, G., Sacks, H., & Schegloff, E. A. (1987). Notes on laughter in the pursuit of intimacy. In G. Button & J. R. E. Lee (Eds.), *Talk and social organization* (pp. 152–205). Clevedon: Multilingual Matters.

Kelly, M., Svrcek, C., King, N., Scherpbier, A., & Dornan, T. (2020). Embodying empathy: A phenomenological study of physician touch. *Medical Education, 54*(5), 400–407. https://doi.org/10.1111/medu.14040

Lu, J. (2016). Will medical technology deskill doctors? *International Education Studies, 9*(7), 130–134. https://doi.org/10.5539/ies.v9n7p130

Orom, H., Underwood, W. III, Cheng, Z., Homish, L., & Scott, Y. (2018). Relationships as medicine: Quality of the physician–patient relationship determines physician influence on treatment recommendation Adherence. *Health Services Research, 53*(1), 580–596. https://doi.org/10.1111/1475-6773.12629

Peräkyla, A. (2006). Communicating and responding to diagnosis. In J. Heritage & D. W. Maynard (Eds.), *Communication in medical care: Interaction between primary care physicians and patients* (pp. 214–247). Cambridge: Cambridge University Press. https://doi.org/10.1017/CBO9780511607172.010

Pilnick, A. (2008). 'It's something for you both to think about': Choice and decision making in nuchal translucency screening for Down's syndrome. *Sociology of Health and Illness, 30*(4), 511–530. https://doi.org/10.1111/j.1467-9566.2007.01071.x

Pilnick, A. & Zayts, O. (2016). Advice, authority and autonomy in shared decision-making in antenatal screening: The importance of context. *Sociology of Health and Illness, 38*(3), 343–359. https://doi.org/10.1111/1467-9566.12346

Robinson, J. D. (2003). An interactional structure of medical activities during acute visits and its implications for patients' participation. *Health Communication, 15*(1), 27–57. https://doi.org/10.1207/S15327027HC1501_2

Robinson, J. D. (2006). Soliciting patients' presenting concerns. In J. Heritage & D. W. Maynard (Eds.), *Communication in medical care: Interaction between primary care physicians and patients* (pp. 22–47). Cambridge: Cambridge University Press. https://doi.org/10.1017/CBO9780511607172.004

Robinson, J. D., & Heritage, J. (2005). The structure of patients' presenting concerns: The completion relevance of current symptoms. *Social Science & Medicine, 61*(2), 481–493. https://doi.org/10.1016/j.socscimed.2004.12.004

Robinson, J. D., & Stivers, T. (2001). Achieving activity transitions in physician-patient encounters from history taking to physical examination. *Human Communication Research, 27*(2), 253–298. https://doi.org/10.1111/j.1468-2958.2001.tb00782.x

Sacks, H., Schegloff, E. A., & Jefferson, G. (1974). A simplest systematics for the organization of turn-taking for conversation. *Language, 50*(4), 696–735. https://doi.org/10.2307/412243

Schegloff, E. A. (2000). On granularity. *Annual Review of Sociology, 26,* 715–720. https://doi.org/10.1146/annurev.soc.26.1.715

Schegloff, E. A. (2001). Accounts of conduct in interaction: Interruption, overlap, and turn-taking. In J. H. Turner (Ed.), *Handbook of sociological theory* (pp. 287–321). Springer. http://dx.doi.org/10.1007/0-387-36274-6_15

Schegloff, E. A. (2007). *Sequence organization in interaction, Vol. 1. A primer in conversation analysis.* Cambridge: Cambridge University Press. http://dx.doi.org/10.1017/CBO9780511791208

Schegloff, E. A., & Sacks, H. (1973). Opening up closings. *Semiotica, 8,* 289–327. https://doi.org/10.1515/semi.1973.8.4.289

Schegloff, E. A., Jefferson, G., & Sacks, H. (1977). The preference for self-correction in the organization of repair in conversation. *Language, 53*(2), 361–382. https://doi.org/10.1353/lan.1977.0041

Sterie, A-C., Weber, O., Jox, R. J., & Truchard, E. R. (in press). 'Do you want us to try to resuscitate?': Conversational practices generating patient decisions regarding cardiopulmonary resuscitation. *Patient Education and Counseling,* https://doi.org/10.1016/j.pec.2021.07.042. Available online 18 August 2021.

Stewart, M., Brown, J. B., Donner, A., McWhinney, I. R., Oates, J., Weston, W. W., & Jordan, J. (2000). The impact of patient-centered care on outcomes. *The Journal of Family Practice, 49*(9), 796–804.

Stivers, T. (2002). Presenting the problem in pediatric encounters: 'Symptoms only' versus 'candidate diagnosis' presentations. *Health Communication, 14*(3), 299–338. https://doi.org/10.1207/S15327027HC1403_2

Stoeckle, J. D., & Billings, J. A. (1987). A history of history-taking: the medical interview. *Journal of General Internal Medicine, 2*(2), 119–127. https://doi.org/10.1007/bf02596310

Toerien, M., Jackson, C., & Reuber, M. (2020). The normativity of medical tests: Test ordering as a routine activity in 'new problem' consultations in secondary care. *Research on Language & Social Interaction, 53*(4), 405–424. https://doi.org/10.1080/08351813.2020.1785768

Wu, R-J. R. (2016). Turn design and progression: Aiyou in Mandarin conversation. *Chinese Language & Discourse, 7*(2), 210–236. https://doi.org/10.1075/cld.7.2.02wu

6 Lifestyle advice-giving and reception

6.1 Introduction

The contemporary practice for chronic disease has undergone an ideological shift from cure to prevention. Numerous studies have suggested a close relationship between lifestyle and chronic conditions such as obstructive pulmonary disease (Cunningham et al., 2014), coronary heart disease (Malhotra et al., 2017), high blood pressure (Jones et al., 2012), diabetes (Rahati et al., 2014), and cancer (Hermans et al., 2021). For older adults, in particular, a close association between a healthy lifestyle and improvement in chronic conditions has been observed (van Gool et al., 2007). However, with few exceptions (Guassora et al., 2015; Sorjonen et al., 2006), knowledge about the interactional dynamics between health providers and patients regarding lifestyle promotion is scarce. To contribute to the understanding of lifestyle communication in medical encounters, this study examines lifestyle advice-giving and reception activities in routine TCM consultations.

Recent research has suggested the delicacy and challenge in advice-giving (Antaki & Bloch, 2020; Heritage & Sefi, 1992). This is particularly the case when delivering lifestyle advice that indicates a problem in the recipient's behaviors. Despite a growing literature suggesting the effectiveness of lifestyle promotion in health maintenance and disease prevention (Noordman et al., 2010; Shatenstein, 2008), such interventions are not widely observed in different medical encounters. Barriers to successful lifestyle advice delivery include factors such as patient resistance (Barton et al., 2016; Bergen, 2020; Jallinoja et al., 2007), doctors' rushed schedules (Koutoukidis et al., 2018), the relevance of the advice to the problem (Guassora & Baarts, 2010), and patient reluctance to admit a problem in their behaviors (Denvir, 2014).

Other studies focus on the sequential organization of lifestyle advice-giving. These studies understand advice delivery as a 'collaborative construction of a problem' (Guassora et al., 2015, p. 191) and that it is ordinarily instantiated via an adjacency pair sequence (Schegloff, 2007). In their path-breaking study, Sorjonen et al. (2006) advanced our knowledge of the collaborative work on lifestyle advice-giving and reception between doctors and patients during acute visits in Finnish primary care consultations. One significant contribution of their

DOI: 10.4324/9781003161929-6

study is the observation of the association between various interactional features (e.g., the sequential environment and forms of doctors' lifestyle questions, and the design of the patient's responses), participants' understanding of patients' lifestyle (problematic or non-problematic), and the relevance of lifestyle advice. A different finding was reported by Guassora et al. (2015) in a study of preventive consultations in Danish general practice. They reported greater participant engagement in lifestyle advice delivery. In their study, the doctor was active in providing evaluative comments (e.g., support or recommendation) on the patient's current habits when both parties were oriented to the patient's lifestyle as non-problematic. They focused on how patients answer their GP's questions about lifestyle. Guassora suggested a standard interview format in the GP-patient lifestyle question-answer sequence: the patient provides the information, and the doctor assesses the risks of the patient's lifestyle. However, in a substantial minority of their observations, the patient bypassed this format by providing self-evaluation that indicated a problematic orientation toward their lifestyle and thereby anticipated lifestyle advice from the GP. Such heterogeneity in previous findings can be possibly explained, inter alia, by the clinical differences between primary care and preventive care. As Guassora et al. stated, such consultations provide a particular frame for lifestyle consultations. In routine primary care consultations, Bergen (2020) examined advice-giving following the patient's disclosure of behaviors that suggest a problem in their lifestyle. Her findings suggest varying patient responses to doctors' advice pertinent to its implications for diagnosis and treatment.

Despite the difference in research focus among these studies, one commonality in their findings is that lifestyle advice-giving is an activity that usually indexes the speaker's problematic orientation toward the recipient's behaviors and that such orientation usually makes lifestyle advice relevant. In this study, I expand earlier work by examining lifestyle advice-giving and reception in routine TCM encounters, focusing on the locations and forms of lifestyle advice and how the offering of advice accomplishes different institutional and interpersonal tasks. The data presented in this study is similar to that of Bergen's (2020) work: on the one hand, different from acute visits, routine encounters require the doctor to assess chronically ill patients, which might include discussions about their lifestyles (e.g., diet, alcohol consumption, and physical exercise). On the other hand, TCM consultations are guided by a unique belief in holism that addresses disease based on various aspects related to the patient's life.

6.2 The concept of lifestyle

Despite the importance of lifestyle in patient health management, there is no clear-cut conceptualization of lifestyle in the literature. Within medical sociology, it is used to refer to the individual patterns of behavior related to health (Abel, 1991; Grzywacz et al., 2012). In the health communication literature, Johanson et al. (1995, 1996) used a post hoc strategy to define the concept of lifestyle. In their studies, lifestyle in medical discourse reflected various topics, including diet, sleep, exercise, risk behaviors, stress management, and environment. This study uses Johanson et al.'s understanding of lifestyle as an umbrella term to refer to a broad range of individual behaviors that might have either positive or negative impacts on people's health. This understanding of lifestyle is also consistent with what has been described in the RIAS coding framework (see Roter, 1977).

6.3 Lifestyle advice after the formulation of a problem

In support of earlier research, in the present TCM corpora, lifestyle advice-giving might be occasioned by the patient's formulation of a problem. The location of the advice indicates a connection between lifestyle behaviors and the patient's situation, and reflects the doctor's orientation toward the patient's behaviors as requiring change. In other words, for example, lifestyle behaviors are considered a possible cause of the patient's problem. The recommendation of a change in such behaviors naturally occurs as a sequential next action. Consider Extracts 1–4. In Extract 1, the lifestyle advice is provided at line 3 after the patient's turn that indexes a problem. The patient visited the doctor to monitor her long-term cough.

```
(1)  Drink more water
01  DOC:  zuiba  gan  bu  gan
           mouth  dry  not  dry
           Do you feel dry or not in the mouth?

02  PAT:  gan  umm:  haihao
           dry  uhm   okay
           Dry uh:m it's okay.

03  DOC:  yao    duo    he    dian    shui
           need  more  drink  a little  water
           You should drink more water.

04  PAT:  shui wo he    de   duo   de  wo xianzai
           water I drink PRT  a lot PRT I   now
           I drink a lot. As I feel

05         houlong nanguo ma
           throat   uncomfortable interval
           uncomfortable in the throat,

06         yihuier jiu  he    shui
           a while will drink water
           I drink water now and then.

07  (0.9)

08  PAT:  wo zhege hui buhui    he yiqian dong guo shoushu     youguan?
           I  this will won't  to past  have had operation relate
           Would it be possible that my problem relates
           to my earlier operation?
```

The doctor's A-not-A question at line 1 marks a transition to history-taking. The doctor tries to explore possible causes that could explain the patient's ailment and accompanying symptoms. The patient's response indicates a less-than-serious problematic orientation. First, the articulation of *uhm* conveys the patient's uncertainty, unreadiness, and hesitation in preparing her answer. Second, the expression of *haihao* ('okay') conveys some sort of reservation. In Chinese, the word *haihao* is semantically similar to *not bad*. The difference between *hao* and *haihao* is comparable to that between *good* and *okay* in English. Thus, the patient's response makes the advice (line 3) relevant. While suggesting the patient drink more water, the doctor displays her orientation toward the patient's behavior as problematic and needing change. The patient is reluctant to admit her inappropriate behavior and disagreed with the doctor's orientation (line 4). 'I drink a lot, as I feel uncomfortable in the throat, I drink water now and then.'

Interestingly, while the patient mentions a high frequency in her drinking, claiming normality in her behavior, the underlying information conveyed in her turn – that her throat feels uncomfortable – suggests a problem. In other words, the patient's responsive turn rejects both the doctor's orientation and the advice. At this point, both parties work together on sequence closure by forgoing the option to speak (line 7) (Hoey, 2014). The patient's pursuit of other possible reasons that could account for her problem (line 8) consolidates her rejection and non-alignment with the doctor.

In Extract 2, the doctor's advice is offered as an immediate next action to the patient's presentation of his mptoms, albeit implicitly. The patient has chronic gastritis. Prior to line 8, the patient tells the doctor that his stomach and abdominal bloating is much better than before.

```
(2)  Eating less and slower
08  P:  DAOshihou chi xiaqu you yidian   sai[sai]
        sometimes eat down have a little block
        Sometimes when I eat and swallow, a little [blocked]

09  D:                                        [sai]    shiba?
                                              block right
                                              [Blocked] right?

10  P:  ai: shaowei you     yidian
        yep a little have a little
        Ye:p a little.

11  D:  ou  pingshi    dage  ma?
        PRT usually hiccups PRT
        Ou do you hiccup at usual?

12  P:  da
        hiccup
        Yes.

13  D:  chi de    shaoyidian manyidian ne?
        eat PRT    less       slower    PRT
        What if we eat less and slower?
```

```
14  P:  wo chi de   bu   duo   de
        I   eat PRT not  much  PRT
        I don't eat much.
15      pingshi ye   jiu  liang wan fan zheyangzi  yi  wan
        usually just just two   bowl rice this size one bowl
        Usually just two bowls of rice, two bowls of this size.
16  D:  yao   shao shi duo  can
        need less eat more meals
        You should have small frequent meals.
17      wei     shi kao     yang de ou
        stomach is  rely on care PRT PRT
        You need to take good care of your stomach.
18  P:  en
        mmm
        Mmm.
```

The patient's telling of his symptoms (lines 8–10) is hearable as having a negative import, indicating a problem with his stomach. Thereafter, the organization
of the doctor's question displays some granularity (Schegloff, 2000). At line 11,
after minimally receiving the patient's information (Wu, 2004), the doctor immediately adds a second TCU with a yes/no symptom-specific inquiry (Heritage
& Robinson, 2006b), which serves a range of interactional purposes. First, it
announces an activity transition (Robinson & Stivers, 2001) from patient-directed
problem presentation to doctor-directed next-action. Second, the design of the
question indexes the doctor's understanding of a possible association between the
patient's reported symptom (feeling blocked in the stomach) and the symptom
indicated in the doctor's inquiry (hiccups). The doctor is doing the confirmation
or disconfirmation of different symptoms for diagnosis. Third, the formulation
of the doctor's question reflects the doctor's alignment with the patient's problematic orientation.

Upon patient confirmation (line 12), the doctor produces a secondary inquiry,
adding particular details (line 13). While the doctor's secondary inquiry can be
taken as a further pursuit – from one level of granularity to another – it is also
possible that the underlying implication indexed in the inquiry ('eating less and
slower') indicates a problem in the patient's behavior. In other words, the doctor's
turn at line 13 could be both a question and advice. In response to the doctor's
dual orientation, the patient claims normality of his behavior (line 14), rejecting
both the problematic orientation and the advice. While a preferred next action
to the patient's rejection might be an agreement with the patient's behavior as
appropriate or a departure from the current topic, the doctor proceeds with her
problem orientation (lines 16–17) and makes it more pronounced via imperatives.
'You should have small frequent meals.' In that sense, the doctor's advice-
giving also displays granularity. On the first level, the doctor designs her advice
in question format, which is more indirect and less forceful. The design of the
advice makes patient confirmation and disconfirmation relevant. On the second

level, the advice is offered more straightforwardly, making patient acceptance or non-acceptance relevant. The doctor's pursuit of patient acceptance is further pronounced immediately in the second TCU of her turn at line 17, building patient knowledge on the importance of healthy lifestyles. Rather than directly rejecting the doctor's advice, the patient indicates agreement with the minimum acknowledgment token *emm*.

Unlike Extracts 1 and 2, where the patient rejects a problem in their behavior, the patient in Extract 3 admits his unhealthy behavior. He is also aware of the association between the behavior and the problem. Yet, he refuses to make a change. In Extract 3, the patient visited the doctor to monitor his asthma. He had recently taken a diagnostic test. Prior to line 1, the doctor asks the patient to show her his previous reports.

```
(3) Cannot quit smoking
01  P: jiu zhege qita    dou haihao
        just this others all good
        Just this one, all the others are good.
02  (0.8)
03  P: zhege keneng    gen chouyan you    guanxi
        this probably   to  smoking have  matter
        Probably, smoking matters.
04  D: na   ni buhao    buyao chouyan de    a?
        then you why not don't smoking PRT PRT
        Then why don't you quit smoking?
05  P: e:   bu chou   zuo budao
        uhm no smoke do   cannot
        Uh:m I cannot make it.
06  D: shenme jiao zuo budao
        what    mean do cannot
        What do you mean you cannot make it?
07  P: wo > zuo budao zuo budao<
        I    do  cannot do cannot
        I > cannot make it, cannot make it <
08      chouyan YOU    guanxi
        smoke    have   matter
        Smoking matters.
09      xiang zhezhong chouyan shi 0 zhi 10
        like  this kind smoke  is  0 to  10
        For this one, it is ranged between 0 to 10 for smokers,
10      bu chouyan shi 0 zhi 5
        no  smoke  is  0 zhi 5
        and 0 to 5 for non-smokers.
11      na   wo dehua 10 hai meiyou shang
        then I case   10 still no    to
        In my case, it is below 10,
```

```
12      shuoming shi chouyan  de guanxi
        suggest  is  smoke    PRT matter
        therefore smoking matters.
13      jiu yijing     bu he    le
        wine already   no drink PRT
        No wines already.
14  D:  jiu yijing bu he le
        wine already no drink PRT
        No wines already,
15      juede zai bu chouyan mei fa      zuoren    le
        feel  more no smoke   no  method be human PRT
        feel that you cannot be human if no smoking as well.
16  P:  ai JIUSHI JIUSHI
        yep right  right
        Yep RIGHT RIGHT.
```

In line 3, the patient produces a candidate diagnosis (Stivers, 2002) of his diagnostic test report, building his reason for the current visit. The claim is heavily assertive: the use of 'just' and 'all the others' displays the patient's certainty about his condition, which is not unexpected as the diagnostic test report normally indicates abnormalities by adding an arrow (either upward or downward) to the left of the item. After 0.8 seconds of silent report reading, the patient breaks the silence by building a connection between his behavior (smoking) and his condition (line 3). In other words, the patient admits his behavior as being unhealthy, making advice-giving relevant. In response to the patient's self-admitted problematic behavior, the doctor builds her advice in her question 'Why don't you quit smoking?' The doctor's turn at line 4 is certainly not heard as a question asking for the reason, but rather, suggesting the patient take an action. The patient's articulation of hesitation (*uh:m*) displays his unreadiness and difficulty, laying the ground for his rejection (line 5). Yet, the patient's rejection is not understood by the doctor, who seeks explanations (line 6). It is also likely that by inviting explanations, the doctor pursues further advice-giving by exploring possible barriers that affect the patient's behavioral change. In response, the patient provides an extensive explanation (lines 7–13). The patient starts with a repetition of his rejection, thereby consolidating his non-acceptance of the advice. Notably, his explanation is delayed in six lines. The patient adds between his rejection and his explanation (line 13) an extensive description of his problem and interpretation of the diagnostic test report. In so doing, the patient acknowledges the benefits of not drinking as recommended by the doctor. In that sense, the patient displays his alignment with the doctor in terms of the appropriateness of the advice, thereby acknowledging the doctor's authority. Yet, the patient also indicates non-compliance by suggesting difficulty in changing his behavior (line 13). Here, at this point, the doctor displays a strong emotional alignment. While the patient's explanation 'no wines already' is not hearable as completed, the doctor first repeats his utterance (line 14) and then finishes it with an explication of the emotional stress. In so doing, the doctor displays her understanding and acceptance. Mutual agreement on not changing the behavior is achieved.

In Extracts 1–3, lifestyle advice is initiated by the doctor as a sequential next action to the patient's formulation of a problem. The place of the advice indicates a connection between the problem and the behavior. In Extracts 4 and 5, lifestyle advice is provided as a second pair part to the patient's question. The placement of the patient's question reflects their understanding of lifestyle behaviors as possible causes of or at least be related to their problems. In Extract 4, the patient was considered to have chronic bronchitis. Prior to line 1, the patient tells the doctor that he always feels uncomfortable in his throat.

```
(4) A healthy diet
01 P: wo jiu  shi yanhou duzhu houlong shaya
      I   just am  throat stuck throat  hoarse
      I got stuck in the throat, and my sound was hoarse
02 D: en
      mmm
      Mmm.
03 P: zhege he yinshi shi bushi ye   you    guanxi?
      this  to diet   yes not  also have connection
      does diet matter or not?
04 D: na kending   de    a
      then sure     PRT PRT
      That's for sure.
05    henduo jibing  DOU shi chi chulai de
      a lot  disease all is  eat out    PRT
      Many diseases are caused by an unhealthy diet.
06    women shuo yao qingdan yinshi ou
      we    say  need light   diet   PRT
      It is said that a healthy diet is light.
07    nianji da le gengjia de lei    ou
      age    old PRT more    PRT PRT PRT
      This is particularly for the aged.
08 P: wo zongyao chi huncai de    a
      I    have to eat meat     PRT PRT
      I have to eat meat.
09    guang baicai    doufu KENDING  buxing   de a
      only vegetable tofu definitely not work PRT PRT
      Vegetables and tofu only DEFINITELY doesn't work
10 D: mei shuo bu rang ni  chi
      not say  not let you eat.
      I am not saying that you cannot eat meat.
11    jiu shi pengren fangshi
      just is cook    approach
      It's just about how you cook the food,
```

```
12      ni   shao dian    you a  shenme de
        you  less a little oil PRT what   PRT
        like you can add less oil,
13      wanshang me    buyao chi tai youni de
        evening  PRT   don't eat too oily  PRT
        and avoid foods that are too oily in the evening.
14  P:  ou   haode
        PRT  okay
        ou okay.
15  D:  ai:  lai   shetou kan yixia
        yep  come  tongue see PRT
        Ye:p come and show me your tongue.
```

The patient's question seeking lifestyle advice (line 3) is raised immediately after the formulation of a problem, indicating his understanding of a possible connection between diet and health. Here, the patient's question invites an answer from the doctor, making advice-giving relevant. The doctor takes up the patient's invitation and offers advice in detail (lines 4–7). She first confirms the patient's understanding and then consolidates that understanding by claiming a universal connection between diet and different diseases. In so doing, the doctor highlights the importance of diet in explaining health. The advice relevant to the patient's question is offered at line 6 and consolidates at line 7. By arguing for a 'particularity' of the aged, the doctor strengthens the importance of a healthy diet for the patient. While patient acceptance is not achieved (lines 8–9), the doctor reformulates her advice. She first corrects the patient's understanding (line 10), thereby agreeing with the patient's behavior. Then the doctor explicates the particular aspects of dietary habits that might affect the patient's health (line 11–13). Upon patient acceptance (line 14), the doctor announces a shift to a physical examination.

A similar pattern can be seen in Extract 5, where the doctor's advice is offered as a response to the patient's question. In Extract 5, the patient had gout. He came to visit the doctor to monitor his condition. He had taken medication for a while. Prior to line 1, the patient tells the doctor that he is becoming much better.

```
(5) Outdoor or indoor exercises
01  P:  jiu   shi haishi you yidiandian zhong
        just  is  still  have a little   swollen
        It's still a little swollen,
02      pa    louti haishi you   dian   tong de
        climb steps still  have a little pain PRT
        it's still painful when I climb the steps.
03  D:  hai zhong      lei
        still swollen  PRT
        It's still swollen.
```

```
04  P:  um   yisheng a    nage piaoling ou
        umm  doctor   PRT that  purine   PRT
        Umm doctor for the purine,

05          chule      yinshi yao  zhuyi
            apart from diet   need watch
            apart from watching the diet,

06          hai     yao zhuyi shenme  a?
            still need watch  what    PRT
            what else shall I pay attention to?

07  D:  yao   duo duanlian
        need more exercise
        More exercises.

08          xiang ni xianzai dehua me keyi SHIdang
            like  you now    case  PRT can  appropriate
            In your current situation, you can APPropriately

09          yundong    yixia
            exercise   PRT
            take some exercises

10  P:  huwai       ou?
        outdoor     PRT
        Outdoor?

11  D:  zhege huwai  haishi shinei me zuihao me huwai
        this  outdoor or     indoor PRT best   PRT outdoor
        Outdoor or indoor, best outdoor.

12          dui ni  xinfei         ye  hao   de
            for you heart and lung also good  PRT
            It's good for your heart and lungs.

13  P:  ou
        PRT
        ou

14  D:  qita zhengzhuang meiyou lou?
        other symptoms   no     PRT
        No other symptoms?
```

After suggesting an improvement in his condition (data not shown), the patient presents a symptoms-only description of his problem (lines 1–2). The doctor aligns with the patient by repeating the patient's turn ('it's still swollen'), suggesting it is not a recent discovery. In response to the doctor's explanation, the patient minimally indicates acceptance at line 8. Immediately after that, he raises his concern about lifestyle behaviors as if they were related to his problem (lines 4–6). 'Apart from watching the diet, what else shall I pay attention to?' The placement of the question reflects the patient's orientation toward lifestyle behaviors as accounting for his problem. The doctor's advice-giving thereafter (lines 7–12) corresponds to such an orientation and confirms the patient's understanding. While patient acceptance is achieved, the doctor announces a shift back to the physiological agenda of the interaction (line 14), indicating a closing of the current sequence.

6.4 Lifestyle advice after diagnosis

There are some instances when lifestyle advice is given after diagnosis and in close proximity to the patient's telling of their symptoms. In such an environment, the advice is usually formulated either as a pronouncement or a suggestion related to treatment (Stivers et al., 2018). In Extract 6, the patient visited the doctor to monitor her high blood pressure. Prior to the conversation, the doctor solicits patient information on a number of issues, including sleep, bowel movement, and blood cell indices.

```
(6)  Kidney deficiency
01  D:  ni zhege TIZHI            a: (.)[zonggui shi: tut
        you this body constitution PRT after all    be: tut
        Your BODY CONSTITUTION is (.) [after all tut,

02  P:                     [ei
                      [yes

03  D:  pian han  de   ti  xu   de (.)
        more cold PRT body weak PRT
        cold and deficient (.)

04      ti    xu   shen  xu
        body weak kidney deficiency
        a deficient body, a deficient kidney

05  P:  ↑ga(.)sanyuefen kaishi chi   qi chi DAO  xianzai de lei
        then  March   start   eat since eat till now     PRT PRT
        ↑I have started taking the medication from March TILL now.

06  D:  suoyi ni >BUSHI< ni-ni  jiu  shi shenme ne(.)
        so    you no    you you just is  what  PRT
        So you >no< you-you're just what (.)

07      ni zhege tizhi            a >leng de dongxi<
        you this body constitution PRT cold PRT stuff
        Given your body constitution, > cold stuff <

08      YIDIAN   dou peng bu lai
        a little all touch no PRT
        you cannot eat AT ALL.

09  P:  leng  a
        cold PRT
        Cold?

10  D:  ↑LENG de dongxi(.)uh:m tian   de dongxi shao chi
          cold PRT stuff   uhm  sweet PRT stuff less eat
        ↑ COLD stuff (.) uh:m eat fewer sweets.
```

At the beginning of this extract, the doctor produces a plain assertion (Peräkylä, 2006) of the patient's disease (lines 1–4). A recurrent theme in the doctor's diagnostic statement is a deficient body. In TCM, the concept of *deficiency* or *deficiency syndrome* is used to 'categorize the patients as lacking some specific element' (Chien et al., 2012, p. 204). According to Chien et al. (2012), patients with any deficiency syndrome might experience similar symptoms as fatigue in WM. In response to the doctor's diagnosis, the patient challenges the doctor by suggesting that she has taken medication for three consecutive months (line 5). The high-pitched onset (Couper-Kuhlen, 2001) and the intonated temporal reference ('TILL') are hearable as expressing doubt about either the doctor's diagnosis or the effects of her previous treatment. The doctor's advice is provided at lines 6–8. Using the *suoyi*-prefaced structure (similar to the *so*-prefaced structure in English), the doctor builds a connection between the diagnosis and the advice. The placement of the advice might also suggest the doctor's orientation toward the recommended behavior as an alternative treatment option to the patient's problem. Interestingly, the prefacing of the connective *suoyi* in introducing the advice (line 6) might reflect the doctor's orientation toward the patient's complaint or challenge as a side sequence to the main course of diagnosis and advice-giving (Wang, 2020). In other words, the doctor announces a return back to the previous agenda of diagnosis, making advice-giving relevant.

While offering the advice, the doctor highlights the importance of avoiding cold foods (lines 6–8). Using imperatives, the advice is formulated as a pronouncement (Stivers et al., 2018), strengthening the force of the advice. The pronouncement is given with no invitation of patient acceptance. In other words, the doctor asserts full agency and authority (Heritage, 2021) over the advice with which the patient shall comply. As a response to the doctor's pronouncement, the patient repeats the advice to confirm understanding. The doctor then repeats the advice (line 10), and adds in the second TCU her secondary pronouncement. Thereafter, the doctor and the patient engage in extensive lifestyle advice-giving (data not shown).

A similar pattern is presented in Extract 7. In Extract 7, the patient came for breast swelling. She had uterine fibroids. Prior to line 1, the patient tells the doctor that her menstrual cycle ended quite a few years earlier. The doctor's extensive advice-giving emerges at line 5 immediately after her diagnostic statement.

```
(7) Watch your diet
01 D: you   shihou    hui  you     dian     zhangtong ou
      have sometimes will have a little  swollen    PRT
      Sometimes you feel swollen?

02 P: en
      umm
      Umm.

03 D: zhege keneng   shi yinwei   ni   jisu   shuiping da
      this probably is because you hormone level    high
      This is probably caused by your high hormone level.
```

```
04    ta zhuyao shi gen cijisu   you     guanxi  de  ou
      it mainly is  to estrogen have relation PRT PRT
      It is mainly related to estrogen level
05    name ni de   hua  ne jiu  shi (.)
      so  you PRT case PRT just is
      So in your case, just
06    ZHUyao          me: yige jiu  shi
      Most important PRT one  just is
      most importantly, one thing is that
07    chi dongxi de   hua  yao ZHUYI   ou
      eat things PRT case need careful PRT
      you need to WATCH your diet
08    shiyong fengjiao fenghuangjiang zhezhong dongxi
      eat     propolis royal jelly    this kind food
      foods such as propolis and rolyal jelly
09    BUyao duo   chi ou
      don't much eat PRT
      don't eat too much
10    haiyou       baokuo youxie ejiao            zhezhong
      in addition include some  donkey-hide gelatin this kind
      and also foods such as the donkey-hide gelatin
11    jinliang           shenzhong ou
      as far as possible careful    PRT
      You need to be careful as far as possible
12 P: ou
      PRT
      ou
13 D: dui(.)  dou yao shenzhong ou
      right   all need careful  PRT
      Right (.) you need to mind all of these foods.
```

Instead of describing the patient's situation as a fact, the doctor provides a diagnosis with reference to the evidence (Peräkylä, 2006). 'This is probably caused by your high hormone level. It is mainly related to estrogen level' (line 4). In so doing, the doctor provides evidence (high hormone level) and offers an explanation (estrogen level) regarding the course of the disease. More importantly, the naming of the cause builds the case for the lifestyle advice in her immediate next TCU at line 5. Using the connective 'so', the doctor indicates a causative connection between her prior action and the recommended behaviors (Schiffrin, 1987). In that sense, a modification of behavior works as a treatment option for the patient's problem. The use of 'so' also projects a transition of activities from diagnosis delivery to advice-giving, marking a boundary within the sequence (Raymond, 2004).

In the extensive turn of advice-giving, the doctor provides clear guidance on dietary behavior by naming different types of foods that should not be eaten.

Yet, the way the doctor designs her advice is different from Extract 6. Here, while the advice is hearable as pronouncements with the imperative form of the utterance (lines 7, 9, 11), the advice is mitigated. By saying 'don't eat too much', the doctor makes her advice less serious and more acceptable. Upon the patient's minimal acceptance (line 12), the doctor indicates agreement and consolidates her advice.

6.5 Lifestyle advice in closing-relevant environments

One particular place where lifestyle advice-giving emerges in the TCM corpora is the closing-relevant environment. It is co-designed (e.g., both parties have the right to initiate the topic) and mutually aligned as the last activity that makes the terminal exchange (Schegloff and Sacks, 1973) relevant. Most importantly, I argue that since the closing phase is the environment where participants raise their 'unmentioned mentionables' (Schegloff and Sacks, 1973), lifestyle advice-giving initiated by the doctor displays their care and concern toward the patient. In this particular place, lifestyle advice-giving accomplishes more than the instrumental tasks of diagnosis and treatment.

In Extract 8, the advice is initiated by the doctor after the completion of several interactional tasks: calling the next patient, printing the prescription form, and signing the form, each of which constituted a closing-relevant environment (Robinson, 2001).

```
(8)  Indiscriminate eating
01  ((the sound of the printer))
02  N:  xxx ((calling the next patient))
03  X:  mm
        mm
04  D:  ziji jian    ou
        self concoct PRT
        You will concoct the herbs by yourself right?
05  P:  mm (.) ziji jian    de
        mmm    self concoct PRT
        Mmm (.) I will do it by myself.
06  (0.2)((the doctor signs))
07  P:  xiexie
        thank you
        Thank you.
08  D:  (h)↑ai:ya ni BIE?   LUAN:        chi dongxi
        aiya you don't indiscriminately eat stuff
        (h)↑ai:ya DON'T? eat INDISCRIMINATELY
09      [le(.)wo dou    you    dianer    PA: ni le]
        PRT    I already have a little scare you PRT
        [(.)You've already SCA:RED me]
```

```
09  P:  [↑>HAO wo bu luan              chi le wo ZAI    YE
        okay  I   no indiscriminately eat PRT I never again
        [↑>OKAY. I won't eat indiscriminately, NEVER AGAIN

10      bu luan            chi le wo zhende xiang<]
        no indiscriminately eat PRT I really want
        I will never eat indiscriminately I really want to <]

11      CHOU si wo ziji   zhen  d- heheh heheh
        slap die I myself really PRT heheh heheh
        kill myself by SLAPPING over the face. Heheh heheh

12  ((the doctor hands over the signed prescription))

13  P:  xiexie xiexie heheh heheh
        thank  thank  heheh heheh
        Thank you. Thank you. Heheh heheh.

14  ((The patient leaves the room))

15  D:  °(h)eh chou: si ziji°
        heh    slap die self
        °(h)eh kill myself by slapping over the face°
```

The patient experienced frequent urination at night, and his eyes were swollen. In their earlier talk, the patient told the doctor that she recently ate some saffron – a type of flower. In the first half of the extract (lines 1–7), there are several opportunities where the doctor orients toward a possible closing: the sound of the printer, the calling of the next patient, and the doctor's signing the prescription form. The doctor's question on the concocting preference (line 4) is an activity normally observed in TCM consultations as a possible last activity that makes closing relevant. The thanking formulae at line 7 is a possible terminal exchange (Schegloff and Sacks, 1973) extensively documented in the literature (Allwood et al., 2017; Park, 2013; West, 2006). Here, the fact that the doctor volunteers lifestyle advice (line 8) in a closing-relevant environment reflects her orientation toward taking the closing as the last opportunity to raise her final concerns. By giving lifestyle advice, the doctor indicates a connection between lifestyle behaviors and the patient's health, accomplishes lifestyle promotion, and shows her stance toward the patient as a person (Lenz & Monagham, 2011). The articulation of the sigh with high pitch and intensity, the intonated negation toward future behavior, and the emotional disclosure (line 9) display the doctor's care for the patient. In that sense, the doctor's advice can also be heard as a critique or disagreement, indicating the patient's behavior as problematic, which, however, was formulated in a less threatening manner. Here, the critique shall be read positively. Instead of putting blame on the patient, the critique builds doctor–patient rapport. 'You've already SCA:RED me.' The doctor's emotional disclosure of scary conveys intimacy and friendliness.

Also notable here is the sigh-prefaced turn (line 8). The doctor's prebeginning sigh (a term used by Hoey, 2014 to describe those appearing before the recognizable onset of a turn) is affectively negative, possibly hearable, inter alia, as disappointment, worry, and fear. Unlike Hoey's (2014) observation, rather than forewarning a dispreferred response, the prebeginning sigh at line 8 forecasts the valence of the response as positive and forestalls a dispreferred response. In so designing, the advice/critique makes patient acceptance relevant. In response, the patient aligns with the doctor both instrumentally and interpersonally. At the instrumental level, the patient explicitly pronounces an understanding of her behavior as problematic and promised a change of behavior. At the interpersonal level, the patient responds with a sincere admission of her behavior as being problematic. '> ↑ OKAY. I won't eat indiscriminately, NEVER AGAIN. I will never eat indiscriminately; I really want < kill myself by SLAPPING over the face. Hehe hehe.' The high-pitched agreement and reification of regret indicate the patient's acceptance of the doctor's advice. The patient's turn has a joke-like quality, and the reification of guilt works like the punchline. Certainly, the patient will not kill herself by slapping her face hard. Instead, the reification serves as an admission of problematic behaviors and an acknowledgment of the advice. The patient's turn-final laughter (line 11) reflects her orientation toward affiliation and relationship building (Fatigante & Orletti, 2013; West, 1984). This orientation extends to line 13, where, after the doctor's closing invitation (i.e., handing over a homeopathic prescription, see Ten Have, 2006), the patient agrees with the doctor in closing the current encounter by showing gratitude. Finally, the joke and the laughter successfully invite the doctor's alignment and reciprocation (Haakana, 2002), evidenced by the affiliated laughing with (Glenn, 2003) and the repetition of the joke (line 15).

In Extract 9, the patient had deficiency syndrome. The doctor's initiation of lifestyle advice is offered after the calling of the next patient, functioning as a take-home note and the last activity of the current consultation.

```
(9) Spicy foods
01  ((The doctor prints the prescription.))
02  D: zai jia  limian ni shaocai de shihou
       at  home inside you cook  PRT when
       When you cook at home,
03     xiang zhezhong  hujiao a  shenme dongxi
       like  this kind pepper PRT such   things
       things such as pepper
04  P: buyao fang a?
       don't add  PRT
       Don't add to the dish?
05  D: keyi chi
       can  eat
       You can.
06  P: keyi chi a?
       can  eat PRT
       I can?
```

```
07 D: keyi chi (.) hujiao ye   keyi chi
       can  eat       pepper also can  eat
       You can (.) you can also eat pepper

08     yidiandian  la   meiyou guanxi
       a little    spicy no   matter
       A small amount matters not.

09 P: ou
      PRT
      Ou.

10 D: yangrou
      mutton
      Mutton

11 P: = yangrou wo bu chi
         mutton  I  no eat
      = I don't eat mutton.

12 D: niurou
      beef
      Beef

13 P: yangrou niurou wo DOU  buyao chi
      mutton  beef    I  both don't eat
      BOTH mutton and beef, I don't like.

14 D: ou   dou bu chi
      PRT both no eat
      Ou, you eat none of them

15    na   mei banfa le
      then no method PRT
      then I have no solutions.

16 P: buxihuan zhege weidao
      dislike  this  flavor
      I'm not too fond of the flavor.

17    LA    keyi chi yidian wo daoshi
      spicy can  eat some   I  instead
      Instead, if I can eat some spicy foods, I would be

18 D: wei         la yidiandian
      a little spicy a little
      A little spicy, a little.

19 P: ou haode
      PRT okay
      Ou okay.

20 D: buyao chi de  xilihuala    de
      don't eat PRT onomatopoeia PRT
      Not too spicy that makes you cry and your nose running.
```

((more discussions on spicy foods are omitted))

```
24 ((The doctor hands the prescription to the patient))
```

```
25 P: en    hao xiexie
       mmm okay thank you
       Mmm, okay, thank you.
```

Extract 9 illustrates an active co-construction of lifestyle advice in TCM closings. The patient had some deficiency syndromes. His hands were always cold, particularly in winter. The doctor consolidates him to have a problem with blood circulation. The printing of the prescription indicates the doctor's orientation toward the accomplishment of core institutional tasks. While it would be appropriate to close the encounter and send the patient off, the doctor takes the opportunity to promote a healthy lifestyle. Most importantly, the advice is provided in detail. Her first advice on adding seasonings (lines 3–8) is quickly accepted by the patient. In her subsequent turns, the doctor continues to specify a variety of foods (pepper, chili, mutton, and beef) that are recommended. Note that all these foods have hot properties. Thus the offering of lifestyle advice before closing the encounter serves multiple interactional tasks. First, it functions as a take-home note of some unmentioned mentionables. Advice on how to eat appropriately was not provided in the doctor and patient's prior conversations. Yet, such information could be important for the patient given his deficiency syndromes. Second, the doctor displays her care to the patient by advising on the patient's dietary behaviors before he leaves. Unlike advice-giving in the first two environments (i.e., after the formulation of a problem and diagnosis), where the advice naturally emerges as a sequential next action, advice-giving in the last minute of the encounter after the completion of core institutional tasks, displays the doctor's mutual orientation toward health promotion and interpersonal care.

Extract 9 also differs from Extract 8 where the doctor's advice indicates a problem in the patient's lifestyle behaviors, building a causative connection between the patient's situation and the advice. In other words, the doctor's advice in Extract 8 functions as a treatment for the patient's problem. However, in Extract 9, the advice is provided as a supplement to the biomedical treatment of the problem. In this sense, the advice accomplishes both interpersonal and institutional tasks related to the medical encounter. Similarly, the patient's showing of gratitude (line 25) after the doctor's handing of the prescription could be a thankful appreciation for both the interpersonal care and institutional cure that he receives.

We see one more instance where the doctor initiates lifestyle advice with a non-problematic orientation toward the patient's behavior in Extract 10. In Extract 10, the patient recently had a loss of appetite.

```
(10) Appropriate amount of exercises
01 D: zhege hen   man  de  yao  deng yixia
       this  very slow PRT need wait  PRT
       This is very slow, you need to wait for a while.
02     xia yige xian
       next one first
       Next one first.
```

```
03  ((The doctor calls the next patient.))
04  D:  ni ziji pingshi keyi    shidang      duanlian yixia ou
        you own usually can    appropriately exercise PRT   PRT
        You can do some appropriate amount of exercises
        at the usual time.
05      meitian  zuo zhe  ye  bu   hao de
        everyday sit PRT also not  good PRT
        Sitting there every day is not good.
06  P:  wo jiu   he tamen tiao tiaowu daoshihou
        I  just and they  dance dance sometimes
        Sometimes I dance with others.
07      zouzou shenme de
        walk   such   PRT
        and take a walk, such like that.
08  D:  dai          jian     de ou?
        on behalf of concoct PRT PRT
        You prefer we concoct the herbs for you?
09  P:  ai
        yep
        Yep.
10  D:  hao   le
        okay PRT
        Okay.
11  P:  xiexie        yisheng ou
        thank you    doctor  PRT
        Thank you, doctor.
12  D:  ai
        yep
        Yep.
```

The doctor's comment on the slow speed of the printing machine functions as an explanation for her calling of the next patient to prepare (lines 1–3), indicating her orientation toward a possible closing of the current consultation. The doctor does not turn to the next patient but instead proceeds with the current patient by giving lifestyle advice. In line 4, the doctor suggests the patient get regular exercise in an appropriate amount. Compared with the advice given in Extract 8 on dietary behavior, the doctor's advice here is more general and universal. It was not specifically designed as either a cause or a treatment of a problem. Rather, the advice on getting regular exercise can work for everyone. The patient reciprocates the doctor's advice by indicating her behavior as healthy. 'Sometimes I dance with others and take a walk, such like that.' The patient claims the normality of her behavior. In response to the patient's no-problem orientation, the doctor announces a topic shift from lifestyle advice-giving to concocting preference, making closing relevant. While it is possible that the doctor considers regular exercise would be helpful for the patient's condition, it is also likely that the doctor indicates her care for the patient by offering general advice about the patient's lifestyle. In addition, the initiation of the advice in an environment where the prescription is being printed slowly and where the next patient is called to get ready, indicates the doctor's orientation toward lifestyle advice-giving as a time filler. After the prescription is printed, the doctor signs and hands it to the patient (line 10), indicating a possible pre-closing (Schegloff & Sacks, 1973).

While Extracts 8–10 present instances where lifestyle advice is initiated by the doctor, the next two extracts illustrate the sequences where the patient take the initiative in seeking lifestyle advice. In such instances, the patient indexes their understanding of lifestyle behaviors as possible impediments to their conditions. In Extract 11, the patient had chronic gastritis.

```
(11) Cold body constitution
01  ((The doctor calls the next patient.))
((Lines omitted))

07  (0.8)
08  P: yisheng  wo wei       bu    hao
        doctor   I  stomach not  good
        Doctor, my stomach is not working properly,

09     shenme dongxi bu   hao chi de   a?
        what   things not fine eat PRT PRT
        which foods should be avoided?

10  D: zhang QI de dongxi LENG de dongxi (.) shao chi
        bloat qi PRT stuff cold PRT stuff      less eat
        Food that makes you feel bloated and COLD food (.) eat less.

11  P: yangrou bu hao chi de   ou?
        mutton  no fine eat PRT PRT
        I cannot eat mutton ou?

12  D: yangrou: SHAO chi dian      keyi de  keyi  de
        mutton    less eat a little fine PRT fine  PRT
        Mutton: not too much would be fine, it's fine.

13     ni      zhiyao   chi le bu    nanshou
        you as long as  eat PRT not uncomfortable
        As long as you don't feel uncomfortable after that,

14     ni   jiu keyi chi
        you just can eat
        you can eat it.

15     yinwei  ni  zhe    ren    pian han  de
        because you this person more cold PRT
        Because your body constitution is cold,

16     yangrou haishi dui ni   bucuo de
        mutton  is      for you good PRT
        mutton would be good for you.

17  P: ou
        PRT
        Ou.
```

```
18  D: danshi ni buneng   chi TAI duo
       but     you cannot eat too much
       But you can't eat too much,
19     chi xiaqu bu xiaohua
       eat  down not digest
       you can't digest it.
20  P: en (.) jiu  ying   chi xiaqu bu xiaohua
       mmm     just manage eat down   not digest
       Mmm (.) I won't be able to digest with that much.
21  D: ai: dui   de
       yep right PRT
       Ye:p right.
22     suoyi ni   yao  shao chi yidian    ou
       so    you  need less eat a little PRT
       So, you need to eat less.
23  P: en    xiexie
       mmm thank you
       Mmm, thank you.
```

After calling to the next patient to get ready (line 1), the doctor and the patient exchange information on the patient's concocting preference and how the herbs should be delivered to the patient (lines omitted). The conversation then moves into silence (line 7), indicating that neither party had particular issues to raise. These activities constitute a closing-relevant environment. The patient's question at lines 8–9 indicates her orientation toward diet as her last concern. The question consists of two parts: the first part describes her problem, and the second part is the question. The foregrounding of the problem reflects the patient's orientation toward dietary behavior as being accountable for her condition. In addition, the question is designed with a negative valence, reflecting the patient's concern that an inappropriate diet could harm her health. As a response to the patient's question, the doctor provides dietary suggestions (line 10). Yet, the doctor's advice is considered general, in which case the patient pursues further inquiry on specific foods (line 11). Similarly, the patient's secondary question is hearable to have a negative import. In both instances (lines 9 and 11), the patient shows interest in foods that should be avoided rather than foods that are recommended. In that sense, the patient is more attentive to the negative impact of diet on health. The patient's secondary question invokes extensive advice-giving at lines 12–19, with different levels of granularity. When giving advice, the doctor also provides explanations by relating the advice to the patient's condition (lines 15–16), making acceptance relevant. The consultation closes with patient acceptance and her thankful appreciation.

A similar pattern can be seen in Extract 12. The patient's question seeking lifestyle advice reflects his concerns about the negative impact of everyday behaviors on his health conditions. In Extract 12, the patient had constipation.

(12) Selective eating

```
01  D: zhege na    qu fuqian zhege qu na    yao
       this  take to pay     this  to get medicines
       Take this to the cashier, and this to the dispensary.

02  P: ou haode
       PRT okay
       Ou, okay.

03  D: en
       mmm
       Mmm.

04  P: nage yisheng a
       that doctor  PRT
       That, doctor,

05     xiang wo zheyang    ou  chi dongxi jiu shi shuo
       like  I  this kind PRT eat stuff  just is  say
       in my sitation, the diet, that is to say,

06     you mei you shenme dongxi chi bu lai de    a?
       have no have what   stuff  eat no  PRT PRT PRT?
       are there any foods that shall be avoided?

07  D: yi    shanghuo de dongxi (.) CIji       de dongxi
       easy heated   PRT stuff      provoking PRT stuff
       Foods that make you feel heated (.) and foods
       that are PROvoking.

08     xiang lajiao a    shenme de
       like  chili  PRT such   PRT
       Foods such as chili.

09     ni    pingshi chi la    ma?
       you at usual  eat spicy PRT
       Do you eat spicy foods at usual times?

10  P: hen   shao chi de
       very few   eat PRT
       Very infrequently.

11  D: ai
       yep
       Yep.

12  P: wo xianzai jiu suannai chi chi
       I  now     just yogurt eat eat
       Now I eat yogurt.

13  D: ai: suannai hao   de
       yep yogurt  good PRT
       Ye:p yogurt is good.

14  P: en (.) na    xiexie    yisheng
       mmm     then thank you doctor
       Mmm (.) then, thank you, doctor.
```

```
15  D:  en
        mmm
        Mmm.
```

At the beginning of this episode, there are several interactional cues indicative of a possible closing of the encounter: the doctor's guidelines on payment and the dispensing of medicines (line 1), the patient's grateful appreciation (line 2), and the doctor's minimal acknowledgment of the patient's gratitude (line 3). At line 4, using *nage* ('that'), the patient introduces lifestyle advice-seeking as a new referent in a highlighted but less imposing way (Huang, 1999; Wang, 2011). The patient's question on dietary behaviors is designed to have some negative import. One possible explanation is that the patient already knows foods that are good for his health and therefore pursued here foods that are not recommended. Yet, it is also likely that the patient considers a connection between dietary behaviors and his diarrhea. In response, the doctor provides advice on foods that are not good for his health (lines 7–8). Doctor–patient alignment is evident at line 9. The doctor's question on the patient's specific dietary behavior (i.e., eating spicy foods) immediately after her advice on avoiding spicy foods indicates her alignment with the patient's orientation toward a possible connection between diet and diarrhea. The doctor's question is hearable as preferring a disagreement. Therefore, when the patient provides a preferred response, the doctor indicates agreement (line 11). The patient proceeds to give lifestyle information. The articulation of eating yogurt in a descriptive statement (line 12) rather than question reflects the patient's understanding of this behavior as being healthy. The utterance is not designed for an answer. In response, the doctor aligns with the patient's orientation by showing agreement on his dietary behavior. The consultation closes with an exchange of thank you.

Extract 13 presents a unique instance where the consultation closes and resumes by the patient's question seeking lifestyle advice at line 5. The reintroduction of a lifestyle topic reflects the patient's orientation toward lifestyle advice as unmentioned mentionables (Schegloff & Sacks, 1973; West, 2006) in the current interaction.

```
(13) Caterpillar fungus
01  D:  daoshihou keyi  zuoxialai yiqi
        by then   can   sit down   together
        By then, we can sit down together
02      gei zhuren     kan   yixia hao  bu  hao?
        to  director   look  PRT   okay not okay
        and ask the director to take a look, okay?
03  P:  Hao  de  Hao  de  xiexie
        okay PRT okay PRT thank you
        Okay, Okay, thank you.
04  ((The patient left))
```

```
05  P: Yisheng wo chongcao            hao bu hao chi de a?
       doctor   I  caterpillar fungus fine not fine eat PRT PRT
       Doctor, can I eat or not caterpillar fungus?

06  D: chongcao          dehua ni chi de  bu  duo  de  lou?
       caterpillar fungus case you eat PRT not much PRT PRT
       Caterpillar fungus, you don't eat a lot, do you?

07     ouer           chi de lou?
       occasionally eat PRT PRT
       You eat it occasionally, don't you?

08  P: dui
       yes
       Yes.

09  D: zhege yinggai wenti yingxiang bu  da  de
       this  should problem impact    not big PRT
       This should have no big problem < impact.

10  P: bu  da
       not big
       Not big?

11  D: ai
       yep
       Yep.

12  P: hao  de xiexie      yisheng
       okay PRT thank you doctor
       Okay, thank you doctor.

13  D: ai zouhao
       yep bye and safe
       Yep. Bye and safe.
```

The consultation closes at line 4 after the doctor's arrangement of future activities (Robinson, 2001) and the patient's indication of appreciation (lines 1–3). Yet, the patient walks into the consultation room again and raises a lifestyle question, asking the doctor if she could eat caterpillar fungus – a type of health supplement. In TCM, it is considered as having a unique impact on balancing *yin* and *yang* and is, therefore, good for one's health. The place of the question indicates the patient's orientation toward lifestyle behaviors as being important for her health, and therefore should be mentioned. As an answer to the patient's question, the doctor provides advice (lines 6–7). Interestingly, the doctor's advice is implicated in her tag questions: 'Caterpillar fungus, you don't eat a lot, do you? You eat it occasionally, don't you?' The successive articulation of two tag questions, with both positive and negative designs, reflects the doctor's preference for the answer. In other words, the doctor indicates that a small amount and occasional intake would be recommended. Upon patient alignment (line 8), the doctor provides a plain assertion (line 9) and confirms thereafter (line 11). As the patient's final concern is solved, the consultation moves to a closure with a terminal exchange (lines 12–13).

6.6 Summary

In Chapters 3 and 4, we see that TCM consultations feature frequent talk about lifestyle communication and that such discussion can be initiated by both the doctor and the patient. In Chapter 5, we see how diagnostic testing in WM might reveal information on the patient's condition and facilitate diagnosis and treatment. In the present chapter, I show how talk about patients' lifestyles reflects participants' orientations toward lifestyle behaviors as causes and treatments of patients' health conditions. I focus on the activity of advice-giving and discussed three environments where such activity naturally emerges as a sequential next action to the prior action(s). Most importantly, the place of lifestyle advice-giving reflects different understandings of the role of lifestyle activities in understanding patient health. Advice after the formulation of a problem suggests a connection between behaviors and problems. While this understanding is also indexed when advice is introduced after diagnosis, there is also an indication toward behavioral change as a possible treatment plan for the patient's problem. A unique place in the TCM corpora is the closing-relevant environment. I argue that advice-giving in medical closings does not have to indicate a problem in the patient's behaviors, but instead, it promotes health and shows interpersonal care. In my observation, lifestyle advice is an activity that can be initiated by both the doctor and the patient. The analysis presented in this chapter supports the findings of the RIAS study by showing how lifestyle communication constructs the three interactional tasks in medical encounters: understanding patient health, proposing treatment options, and building rapport.

References

Abel, T. (1991). Measuring health lifestyles in a comparative analysis: Theoretical issues and empirical findings. *Social Science & Medicine, 32*(8), 899–908. https://doi.org/10.1016/0277-9536(91)90245-8

Allwood, R., Pilnick, A., O'Brien, R., Goldberg, S., Harwood, R. H., & Beeke, S. (2017). Should I stay or should I go? How healthcare professionals close encounters with people with dementia in the acute hospital setting. *Social Science & Medicine, 191*, 212–225. https://doi.org/10.1016/j.socscimed.2017.09.014

Antaki, C., & Bloch, S. (2020). Advising without personalising: How a helpline may satisfy callers without giving medical advice beyond its remit. *Sociology of Health & Illness, 42*(5), 1202–1219. https://doi.org/10.1111/1467-9566.13088

Barton, J., Dew, K., Dowell, A., Sheridan, N., Kenealy, T., Macdonald, L., Docherty, B., Tester, R., Raphael, D., Gray, L., & Stubbe, M. (2016). Patient resistance as a resource: candidate obstacles in diabetes consultations. *Sociology of Health & Illness, 38*(7), 1151–1166. https://doi.org/10.1111/1467-9566.12447

Bergen, C. (2020). The conditional legitimacy of behavior change advice in primary care. *Social Science & Medicine, 255*, 112985. https://doi.org/10.1016/j.socscimed.2020.112985

Chien, T-J., Song, Y-L., Lin, C-P., & Hsu, C-H. (2012). The correlation of Traditional Chinese Medicine deficiency syndromes, cancer related fatigue, and quality of life in breast cancer patients. *Journal of Traditional and Complementary Medicine, 2*(3), 204–210. https://doi.org/10.1016/S2225-4110(16)30101-8

Couper-Kuhlen, E. (2001). Interactional prosody: High onsets in reason-for-the-call turns. *Language in Society, 30*(1), 29–53. https://doi.org/10.1017/S0047404501001026

Cunningham, T. J., Ford, E. S., Rolle, I. V., Wheaton, A. G., & Croft, J. B. (2014). Associations of self-reported cigarette smoking with chronic obstructive pulmonary disease and co-morbid chronic conditions in the United States. *COPD: Journal of Chronic Obstructive Pulmonary Disease, 12*(3), 281–291. https://doi.org/10.3109/15412555.2014.949001

Denvir, P. (2014). Saving face during routine lifestyle history taking: How patients report and remediate potentially problematic conduct. *Communication & Medicine, 11*(3), 263–274. http://dx.doi.org/10.1558/cam.v11i3.17876

Fatigante, M., & Orletti, F. (2013). Laughter and smiling in a three-party medical encounter: Negotiating participants' alignment in delicate moments. In P. Glenn & E. Holt (Eds.), *Studies of laughter in interaction* (pp. 161–183). London: Bloomsbury. http://dx.doi.org/10.5040/9781472542069.ch-008

Glenn, P. (2003). *Laughter in interaction*. Cambridge: Cambridge University Press. https://doi.org/10.1017/CBO9780511519888

Grzywacz, J. G., Stoller, E. P., Brewer-Lowry, A. N., Bell, R. A., Quandt, S. A., & Arcury, T. A. (2012). Gender and health lifestyle: An in-depth exploration of self-care activities in later life. *Health Education & Behavior, 39*(3), 332–340. https://dx.doi.org/10.1177%2F1090198111405195

Guassora, A. D., & Baarts, C. (2010). Smoking cessation advice in consultations with health problems not related to smoking? Relevance criteria in Danish general practice consultations. *Scandinavian Journal of Primary Health Care, 28*(4), 221–228. https://doi.org/10.3109/02813432.2010.506805

Guassora, A. D., Nielsen, S. B., & Reventlow, S. (2015). Deciding if lifestyle is a problem: GP risk assessments or patient evaluations? A conversation analytic study of preventive consultations in general practice. *Scandinavian Journal of Primary Health Care, 33*(3), 191–198. https://doi.org/10.3109/02813432.2015.1078564

Haakana, M. (2002). Laughter in medical interaction: From quantification to analysis, and back. *Journal of Sociolinguistics, 6*(2), 207–235. https://doi.org/10.1111/1467-9481.00185

Heritage, J. (2021). The expression of authority in US primary care: Offering diagnoses and recommending treatment. In C. Gordon (Ed.), *Approaches to discourse analysis* (pp. 104–122). Washington, DC: Georgetown University Press.

Heritage, J., & Robinson, J. D. (2006b). The structure of patients' presenting concerns: Physicians' opening questions. *Health Communication, 19*(2), 89–102. https://doi.org/10.1207/s15327027hc1902_1

Heritage, J., & Sefi, S. (1992). Dilemmas of advice: Aspects of the delivery and reception of advice in interactions between health visitors and first-time mothers. In P. Drew & J. Heritage (Eds.), *Talk at work: Interaction in institutional settings* (pp. 359–417). Cambridge: Cambridge University Press.

Hermans, K. E. P. E., van den Brandt, P. A., Loef, C., Jansen, R. L. H., & Schouten, L. J. (2021). Alcohol consumption, cigarette smoking and cancer of unknown primary risk: Results from the Netherlands cohort study. *International Journal of Cancer, 148*(7), 1586–1597. https://doi.org/10.1002/ijc.33328

Hoey, E. M. (2014). Sighing in interaction: Somatic, semiotic, and social. *Research on Language and Social Interaction, 47*(2), 175–200. https://doi.org/10.1080/08351813.2014.900229

Huang, S. (1999). The emergence of a grammatical category definite article in spoken Chinese. *Journal of Pragmatics, 31*(1), 77–94. https://doi.org/10.1016/S0378-2166(98)00052-6

Jallinoja, P., Absetz, P., Kuronen, R., Nissinen, A, Talja, M., Uutela, A., & Patja, K. (2007). The dilemma of patient responsibility for lifestyle change: Perceptions among primary care physicians and nurses. *Scandinavian Journal of Primary Health Care, 25*(4), 244–249. https://doi.org/10.1080/02813430701691778

Johanson, M., Larsson, U. S., Säljö, R. & Svärdsudd, K. (1995). Lifestyle in primary health care discourse. *Social Science & Medicine, 40*(3), 339–348. https://doi.org/10.1016/0277-9536(94)e0101-w

Johanson, M., Larsson, U. S., Säljö, R. & Svärdsudd, K. (1996). Addressing lifestyle in primary health care. *Social Science & Medicine, 43*(3), 389–400. https://doi.org/10.1016/0277-9536(95)00403-3

Jones, D. E., Carson, K. A., Bleich, S. N., & Cooper, L. A. (2012). Patient trust in physicians and adoption of lifestyle behaviors to control high blood pressure. *Patient Education and Counseling, 89*(1), 57–62. https://doi.org/10.1016/j.pec.2012.06.003

Koutoukidis, D. A., Lopes, S., Fisher, A., Williams, K., Croker, H., & Beeken, R. J. (2018). Lifestyle advice to cancer survivors: A qualitative study on the perspectives of health professionals. *BMJ Open, 8*(3), e020313. http://dx.doi.org/10.1136/bmjopen-2017-020313

Lenz, T. L., & Monagham, M. S. (2011). Implementing lifestyle medicine with medication therapy management services to improve patient centered health care. *Journal of the American Pharmacists Association, 51*(2), 184–188. https://doi.org/10.1331/JAPhA.2011.10169

Malhotra, A., Redberg, R. F., & Meier, P. (2017). Saturated fat does not clog the arteries: coronary heart disease is a chronic inflammatory condition, the risk of which can be effectively reduced from healthy lifestyle interventions. *British Journal of Sports Medicine, 51*(15), 1111–1112. http://dx.doi.org/10.1136/bjsports-2016-097285

Noordman, J., Verhaak, P., & Van Dulmen, S. (2010). Discussing patient's lifestyle choices in the consulting room: analysis of GP-patient consultations between 1975 and 2008. *BMC Family Practice, 11*, 87. https://doi.org/10.1186/1471-2296-11-87

Park, Y. (2013). Negotiating last-minute concerns in closing Korean medical encounters: The use of gaze, body and talk. *Social Science & Medicine, 97*, 176–191. https://doi.org/10.1016/j.socscimed.2013.08.027

Peräkyla, A. (2006). Communicating and responding to diagnosis. In J. Heritage & D. W. Maynard (Eds.), *Communication in medical care: Interaction between primary care physicians and patients* (pp. 214–247). Cambridge: Cambridge University Press. https://doi.org/10.1017/CBO9780511607172.010

Rahati, S., Shahraki, M., Arjomand, G., & Shahraki, T. (2014). Food pattern, lifestyle and diabetes mellitus. *International Journal of High Risk Behaviors, 3*(1), e8725. https://dx.doi.org/10.5812%2Fijhrba.8725

Raymond, G. (2004). Prompting action: The stand-alone 'so' in ordinary conversation. *Research on Language and Social Interaction, 37*(2), 185–218. https://doi.org/10.1207/s15327973rlsi3702_4

Robinson, J. D. (2001). Closing medical encounters: Two physician practices and their implications for the expression of patients' unstated concerns. *Social Science & Medicine, 53*(5), 639–656. https://doi.org/10.1016/S0277-9536(00)00366-X

Robinson, J. D., & Stivers, T. (2001). Achieving activity transitions in physician-patient encounters from history taking to physical examination. *Human Communication Research, 27*(2), 253–298. https://doi.org/10.1111/j.1468-2958.2001.tb00782.x

Roter, D. L. (1977). *The Roter method of interaction process analysis (RIAS manual).* Baltimore: Johns Hopkins University Press.

Schegloff, E. A. (2000). On granularity. *Annual Review of Sociology, 26,* 715–720. https://doi.org/10.1146/annurev.soc.26.1.715

Schegloff, E. A. (2007). *Sequence organization in interaction. Vol. 1. A primer in conversation analysis.* Cambridge: Cambridge University Press. http://dx.doi.org/10.1017/CBO9780511791208

Schegloff, E. A., & Sacks, H. (1973). Opening up closings. *Semiotica, 8,* 289–327. https://doi.org/10.1515/semi.1973.8.4.289

Schiffrin, D. (1987). *Discourse markers.* Cambridge: Cambridge University Press. https://doi.org/10.1017/CBO9780511611841

Shatenstein, B. (2008). Impact of health conditions on food intakes among older adults. *Journal of Nutrition for the Elderly, 27*(3–4), 333–361. https://doi.org/10.1080/01639360802265889

Sorjonen, M. L., Raevaara, L., Haakana, M., Tammi, T., & Peräkylä, A. (2006). Lifestyle discussions in medical interviews. In J. Heritage & D. W. Maynard (Eds.), *Communication in medical care: Interaction between primary care physicians and patients* (pp. 340–378) Cambridge: Cambridge University Press. https://doi.org/10.1017/CBO9780511607172.014

Stivers, T. (2002). Presenting the problem in pediatric encounters: 'Symptoms only' versus 'candidate diagnosis' presentations. *Health Communication, 14*(3), 299–338. https://doi.org/10.1207/S15327027HC1403_2

Stivers, T., Heritage, J., Barnes, R. K., McCabe, R., Thompson, L., & Toerien, M. (2018). Treatment recommendations as actions. *Health Communication, 33*(11), 1335–1344. https://doi.org/10.1080/10410236.2017.1350913

Ten Have, P. (2006). On the interactive constitution of medical encounters. *Revue Française de Linquistique Appliquée, 11*(2): 85–95. https://doi.org/10.3917/rfla.112.0085

Van Gool, C. H., Kempen, G. I. J. M., Penninx, B. W. J. H., Deeg, D. J. H., & van Eijk, J. T. M. (2007). Chronic disease and lifestyle transitions: Results from the longitudinal aging study Amsterdam. *Journal of Aging and Health, 19*(3), 416–438. https://doi.org/10.1177%2F0898264307300189

Wang, X-Y. (2020). Managing a suspended course of action: A multimodal study of suoyi 'so'-prefaced utterances in Mandarin conversation. *Chinese Language and Discourse, 11*(2), 306–334. https://doi.org/10.1075/cld.20011.wan

Wang, Y. (2011). A discourse-pragmatic functional study of the discourse markers— Japanese *ano* and Chinese *nage*. *Intercultural Communication Studies, 20*(2), 41–61.

West, C. (1984). *Routine complications: Troubles with talk between doctors and patients.* Bloomington: Indiana University Press.

West, C. (2006). Coordinating closings in primary care visits: Producing continuity of care. In J. Heritage & D. W. Maynard (Eds.), *Communication in medical care: Interaction between primary care physicians and patients* (pp. 379–415). Cambridge: Cambridge University Press. https://doi.org/10.1017/CBO9780511607172.015

Wu, R-J. R. (2004). *Stance in talk: A conversation analysis of Mandarin final particles.* Amsterdam: John Benjamins. https://doi.org/10.1075/pbns.117

7   Nonmedical small talk

7.1 Introduction

To date, there have been numerous studies discussing the bigness of small talk in different types of interaction (Holmes, 2000; Hössjer, 2013; Mak, 2019), particularly in medical interactions (Hudak & Maynard, 2011; Maynard & Hudak, 2008; Penn & Watermeyer, 2012; Ragan, 2000). Scholars seem to agree on the value of small talk in satisfying patients' interpersonal needs in medical consultations. However, doctors and patients constantly face the challenge of negotiating interpersonal and instrumental talk given the limited time, the patient loads, and the overarching goal of completing core medical tasks (Beck & Ragan, 1992). This dilemma thus necessitates a reconsideration of the extent to which small talk is appropriate for medical interviews and its functions to accomplish both instrumental and interpersonal tasks. For example, Benwell and McCreaddie (2016) observed that professionals might divert or curtail small talk into extensive troubles-telling in case it might interfere with core instrumental tasks. Otherwise, Maynard and Hudak (2008) noted that health professionals might use small talk to disattend the ongoing instrumental tasks. These findings point to the various functions and status of small talk in medical consultations. This chapter contributes to the literature by examining the functions of small talk in both TCM and WM consultations, focusing on how participants collaboratively engage/disengage in small talk.

Prior studies have suggested various ways in which participants indicate power (Holmes & Stubbe, 2015), one of which is the engagement or disengagement in social conversations that are not directly related to the instrumental talk. In the data to be discussed, the doctor usually has the right to license nonmedical small talk and decide the extent to which talk of this nature is allowed in the here-and-now interaction. The main issue to be explored in this chapter is how doctors and patients engage in small talk and how the treatment of small talk reflects participants' relationships in different encounters. The research questions to be addressed in this chapter are the following:

- Where does small talk occur in TCM and WM encounters?
- How is it interactionally accomplished by participants?

DOI: 10.4324/9781003161929-7

- What are the functions of small talk when placed in different sequential locations?
- How can the treatment of small talk possibly indicate the relationship between the doctor and the patient?

The chapter begins with a review of studies in small talk, particularly in medical contexts. I then analyze small talk in two sequential environments: before patient gloss of their general condition (i.e., in the openings phase of the consultation) and after the printing of the prescription (i.e., in closing-relevant environments).

7.2 Defining small talk

Scholarship on small talk has yielded various definitions. Dictionaries define small talk as unimportant, trivial, and peripheral talk (Schneider, 1988). Early formulations of small talk as a mode of action were developed from Malinowski's conception of phatic communion. The term 'phatic communion' was coined by Malinowski (1923) to describe the function of language as a mode of action instead of a reflection of thought. In his initial interpretation, Malinowski described phatic communion as a form of small talk, the function of which is not for the transmission of thought but rather to achieve companionship. According to Malinowski, this kind of utterance is produced to bind the speaker and the hearer by 'a tie of some social sentiment' (p. 315). In a later edition of this seminal work, Malinowski also borrowed the notion of politeness to explain the function of phatic communion:

> A mere phrase of politeness [...] fulfills a function to which the meaning of its words is almost completely irrelevant. Inquiries about health, comments on weather, affirmations of some supremely obvious state of things – all such are exchanged, not in order to inform, not in this case to connect people in action, certainly not in order to express any thought.
>
> (Malinowski, 1972, p. 313)

Drawing on Malinowski's view, Laver (1975, 1981) characterized small talk as a way to manage interpersonal relationships within the psychosocial realm of interaction. A major contribution of his work is that he reminded us of the indexical nature of small talk in the overarching project of relationship building. In his thoughtful analysis of conversational openings and closings, Laver (1975) posited phatic communion in conversational openings to fulfill a propitiatory function, that is, to prevent or break silence. Laver also noted that when phatic communion emerges in conversational closings, it has a mitigating force so that interlocutors consent and cooperate in terminating the conversation while delivering respect and appreciation. In that sense, phatic communion consolidates interpersonal relationships. According to Laver (1975), a prime function of phatic communion is the 'communication of indexical facts about the speaker's identities, attributes, and attitudes, and that these indexical facts constrain the nature of the particular interaction' (p. 217). In so understanding, Laver points to the relevance and value of small talk to the whole interaction.

While these earlier efforts provide illuminating insights in understanding small talk, a well-rehearsed criticism of such a rigid definition is that it underestimates the various functions of small talk in a broader social context (Coupland, 2000). Studies following the interactional tradition (e.g., social constructionism and ethnomethodology) suggest a context-based approach to evaluate the functions of small talk within the whole interaction. These studies propose that given the fuzzy boundaries between what is socially and institutionally constituted (Roberts 2008), the functions of discourse emerge and change as the conversation flows. For example, Holmes (2000) suggested that small talk may extend along a continuum from the ritualized greeting and parting exchanges to social chitchat, and to some point of the instrumental talk. This porous nature of talk is particularly salient in medical interviews, which feature hybrid modes of talk (Roberts & Sarangi 1999), and these modes can be closely interwoven with each other. Ragan (2000) noted that small talk in women's healthcare encounters is pivotal to achieving instrumental tasks. In fact, Ragan was careful to displace the notion of *small* by the concept of sociable or relational talk. As Coupland et al. (1992) stated,

> The function of particular sequences of talk as phatic or otherwise should not be preconceived. Relevant analytic questions are whether, how, and when talk is oriented to as phatic or not, contingent upon its local sequential placement in particular contextualized episodes and on the momentary salience of particular interactional goals.
>
> (p. 215)

Drawing from insights gained from studies using the interactional approach, this chapter defines small talk as a collaboratively accomplished project, the function of which is context-based rather than being static. Most importantly, how participants attend or disattend to small talk is dependent on and reflective of the interactional norms of different medical practices.

7.3 Small talk at medical openings

Studies have indicated that the opening phase of medical consultations is critical to building patient trust and doctor–patient rapport (Fawole & Rammala, 2021). Prior research suggests that medical encounters normally start with greetings such as *how-are-you* (HAY, Coupland et al., 1992; Heritage & Robinson, 2006; Robinson, 1998; Van der Laaken & Bannink, 2020) before determining the patient's chief complaint. These studies point to two possible interpretations of HAY: as a general inquiry to elicit patient evaluations of their conditions and as a phatic communion (Laver, 1975). Yet, such a phatic or scripted exchange of HAY was only scarcely observed in the present corpora: in 33% of TCM and 5% of WM openings. This finding is at odds with previous research (e.g., Coupland et al.,

Table 7.1 Occurrences of small talk at medical openings and closings

	TCM	WM
Opening	10	2
Closing	27	17
Total number of visits	30	39

1994), suggesting that participants in this study are more oriented to the instrumental agenda of the consultation at the opening phase of a medical encounter. Instead, most of the conversations were opened by the doctor's inquiry to elicit patient concerns or a patient-initiated formulation of a problem. Table 7.1 charts the differences between TCM and WM in relation to the occurrences of small talk at medical openings and closings.

7.3.1 Formulaic sequence of greeting

As Table 7.1 illustrates, small talk emerges more frequently in TCM openings than in WM openings. Most WM consultations opened with core medical talk that directly addresses the instrumental agenda of the consultation. Consider Extracts 1 and 2 – the only two cases in WM encounters that involve a minimum phatic exchange at the opening stage.

```
(1) Non-reciprocated HAY
01  D: nihao
        hello
        Hello.
02  P: wo nage peiyao
        i   that medication refill
        I came for medication refill.
03  D: ou (.) peiyao
        PRT    medication refill
        Ou (.) medication refill.

(2) Respect-delivery addressing
01  P: yisheng
        doctor
        Doctor.
02  D: mmm  zenme bu   hao?
        mmm  how   not  good
        Mmm what's wrong?
```

In both extracts, the opening greeting is disattended. In (1), the doctor starts the consultation with the prototypical *hello*, making a greeting relevant. While a preferred action to the doctor's greeting would be a greeting in return, the patient responds with a pronouncement of her primary concern for the current visit. The patient designs her turn in a way that announces a frame shift from greeting to setting the reason for the visit. The patient's responsive turn thus indicates her orientation toward the current interaction as strictly instrumental. The doctor's affiliation to the patient's stance endorses the legitimacy of core medical talk at this point.

Similarly, in (2), the patient opens the conversation by addressing the doctor, indicating her presence while showing respect to the doctor. The doctor first makes a minimal acknowledgment of the patient's addressing, displaying her realization of the patient's presence. However, immediately in her second TCU, the doctor produces an inquiry about the patient's reason for the visit, making problem presentation relevant. The design of the doctor's turn reflects her orientation toward a frame shift from medical openings to problem presentation. In both cases, the phatic sequence in WM openings starts with the first component being a greeting and the second component being core medical talk.

By contrast, the phatic communion in TCM openings is more extended, with more engaged participation from both the doctor and the patient. Consider Extracts 3 and 4.

```
(3) HAY
01  D: HEI nihao
       hey hello
       HEY hello.
02  P: yisheng
       doctor
       Doctor.
03  D: nihao (.) zuijin:    haihao ba?
       hello     recently   okay    PRT
       Hello (.) you're okay recently?
04  P: um (.) haihao
       mmm     okay
       Mmm (.) okay.
05  D: xiongTONG     a zhe fangmian zenmeyang a?
       breast pain PRT this aspect  how        PRT
       How's your breast PAIN?
```

In (3), the sequence begins with the doctor's greeting. Here, the doctor designs her turn to display familiarity between herself and the patient. The intonated hey before the canonical hello can be heard as indicating surprise, the kind of emotion that is not normally seen between strangers. In other words, the intonated hey suggests acquaintance between the doctor and the patient. In line 2, the patient affiliates with the doctor's action and stance by providing a respect-delivering response (i.e., addressing the doctor). By addressing the doctor, the patient also co-constructs the accomplishment of the presence-acknowledging sequence. Besides acknowledging each other's presence, the greeting sequence can also reveal participants' identities. Here, while the patient's addressing the doctor indicates her respect toward the doctor as the authority in the current interaction, the doctor's intimate greeting mitigates the power asymmetry between conversational parties. Such intimacy extends to lines 3 and 4, where the doctor produced a secondary greeting, followed by an inquiry about the patient's status. Here, the doctor's inquiry can be heard as either a form of phatic communion, similar in its function as the HAY greeting, or a gloss for confirmation (Heritage & Robinson, 2006), making confirmation or disconfirmation relevant (Raymond, 2003). Alternatively, such a gloss might also provide an opportunity for patient elaboration (Pomerantz, 1980). The patient's short response indicates her orientation toward the doctor's inquiry as being phatic and interpersonal. Thus far, the doctor and the patient have co-constructed the interpersonal frame of the current interaction.

```
(4)  HAY-addressing
01  D:  nihao  a
        hello  PRT
        Hello.
02  P:  yisheng    a
        doctor     PRT
        Doctor.
03  D:  ai: nihao
        yep hello
        Ye:p hello.
04  P:  he   haojiu    mei  lai   le
        heh  very long  not  come  PRT
        Heh, it's been quite a while since my last visit.
05  D:  ai: haojiu    mei jian ni   le a
        yep very long  not see  you  PRT PRT
        Ye:p it's been quite a while since I saw you last time
06          zheci       lai    shi:-
            this time  visit  is
            this time you're:-
```

The sequence begins with the doctor's greeting, which is reciprocated with the patient's respect-delivery addressing of the doctor (lines 1–2). In line 3, the doctor first registers acknowledgement of the patient's addressing her and then produces a secondary greeting. While the doctor's first greeting at line 1 can be heard as acknowledging the other's presence, the doctor's secondary greeting in response to the patient's addressing her can be heard as displaying politeness and affiliating. The patient's heh-prefaced statement at line 4 indicates her orientation toward the current interaction as relationship building (Defibaugh, 2018). By suggesting a time gap between the current visit and his last visit, the patient designs his turn in a way that is hearable as a greeting between friends who have not seen each other for a long time. The doctor affiliates with the patient's stance by endorsing the time gap. Thus far, the doctor and the patient display a mutual orientation toward the current interaction as establishing rapport and building a positive doctor–patient relationship, the accomplishment of which makes a shift to instrumental talk relevant (line 6).

In both cases, the opening phatic sequence in TCM encounters features a mutuality in participants' orientation toward the opening phase as an environment where some interpersonal activities will foreground the core medical tasks. I provide one more extract below where the opening phatic sequence is initiated by the patient.

```
(5) Acknowledging the addressing
01  P:  yisheng
        doctor
        Doctor.
02  D:  um   nihao
        mmm  hello
        Mmm hello.
03  P:  wo zuijin    zhege shuimian ou
        i  recently  this  sleep   PRT
        recently I my sleep
04      zuomeng (.) wanshang LAO    zuomeng
        dream       night    always dream
        dream (.) I ALWAYS dream at night.
```

In response to the patient's opening address, the doctor first produces a neutral, minimal acknowledgment token (Gardner, 2001), indicating information reception and acknowledging the patient's presence. Then immediately thereafter, the doctor adds a second TCU in her turn, a greeting, displaying politeness and phaticity. Thus far, the doctor and the patient have co-accomplished a minimal exchange of phatic communion, making frame shift relevant (lines 3–4).

7.3.2 *Social talk at medical openings*

Alternatively, medical openings might involve social talk – talk about some non-controversial' topics (Holmes, 2005, p. 353) such as weather and work. Small talk formulated as such only occurs in TCM encounters. Consider Extract 6:

```
(6) Talk about the weather
01  D:  haoxiang: LEN  qilai le   ai
        seems     cold PRT   PRT  PRT
        seems that it's getting COLD.
02  P:  len qilai↑ ni chuan de SHAO ai [hehe]
        cold PRT   you wear PRT few PRT hhheh
        cold↑ you wear FEW [hhheh]
```

```
03  D:                                        [hehe]
                                             hhheh
                            [hhheh]
04  P:  Wo ne: mei zuo shoushu
        i   PRT not do operation
        I did not take the operation.
```

The sequence begins with the doctor's initiation of talk about the weather, displaying her orientation toward the current interaction as being interpersonal rather than instrumental. The doctor certainly does not intend to comment on the weather change at this point. Instead, the initiation of weather talk can be interpreted as a form of relational talk (Holmes & Woodhams, 2013; Ragan, 2000), functioning as a transition to the instrumental agenda of the encounter. Alternatively, the initiation of a medical encounter with nonmedical social talk could alleviate the seriousness of the encounter, displaying the speaker's friendliness. In line 2, the patient affiliates with the action performed (i.e., talk about non-controversial topics) and the stance indexed (i.e., an orientation toward the interpersonal agenda of the encounter) in the doctor's statement by commenting on the doctor's clothing. Here, the patient designs her turn to display friendliness and intimacy. Thus far, the doctor and the patient have demonstrated a mutual orientation toward social talk as the task of the current interaction. The shared laughter at lines 2 and 3 announces a topic termination (Holt, 2010), displays intimacy (Jefferson et al., 1987), and registers the participants' satisfaction toward the mutual interpersonal orientation, making a frame shift relevant. In line 4, the patient announces a frame shift to the instrumental agenda of the encounter by presenting information related to her medical history (line 4). A more extensive sequence of social talk is presented in Extract 7, where the doctor pursues further the patient's social life by asking about his work after the opening phatic sequence of greetings.

```
(7) Talk about work
01  D:  ni    a: HAOjiu-    liuyuefen-
        you PRT quite long June
        You've been long- June-
02  P:  shi de
        yes PRT
        Yes.
03  D:  BANnian    lou
        half year PRT
        It's been half a year
04      [Bannian    mei chi zhongyao]            lou
         half year no   eat   herbal medicine PRT
        [half a year without Chinese herbal medications?
05  P:  [AI: shi de  shi de ]
        yep yes PRT yes PRT
        Ye:p yes yes.
```

```
06  D:  xianzai  DOU  haihao  ba?
        now      all  okay    PRT
        Is everything okay now?
07  P:  um
        mmm
        Mmm.
08  D:  zuijin:   mang bu  mang?
        recently  busy not busy
        Are you busy or not recently:?
09  P:  xianzai bu zenme mang
        now        not very busy
        not very busy now.
10  D:  keSou a     shenme dou meiyou ou?
        cough PRT   such   all  no    PRT
        no symptoms such as COUgh right?
```

Extract 7 illustrates how work-related talk emerges in the opening phase of medical consultations and how it functions as a transitional device to some serious medical talk. In line 1, the doctor opens the consultation by announcing that she had not seen the patient for quite a while. The temporal reference functions as a support to the doctor's announcement of the time gap. The patient endorses the doctor's recalling of their last visit as correct (line 2). While statements such as 'it's been quite a while since I saw you last' are canonical expressions in Chinese conversations between people who do not see each other regularly, the doctor designs her turn as more than just phatic. The fact that the doctor is able to recall the approximate time of their last visit suggests an intimacy between the conversational parties. It also conveys the doctor's care toward the patient as a person. After the patient's endorsement, the doctor continues her relationship building by reformulating her prior action in a way that integrates small talk and core medical talk, allowing the emergence of her multiple identities: a professional identity whose task is to provide medications to the patient and a social identity whose task is to build rapport. Here, the doctor designs her turn as a 'lamination' (Holmes & Woodhams, 2013, p. 280) of small talk and core medical talk. The patient's responsive turn, the multiple saying of *yes* (Stivers, 2004), targets not only the immediately prior talk but also the entire course of action, the doctor's announcement that she has not seen the patient for a while (lines 1–4). The doctor's mutual orientation extends to her next turn at line 6, which can be heard both as a general inquiry (Heritage & Robinson, 2006) and a phatic communion similar in its function as HAY. In that sense, the doctor leaves the patient with an opportunity to either present her medical concerns or construct interpersonal relationships with the doctor. Yet, the patient foregoes the opportunity by responding with the neutral acknowledgment token *mmm*, proffering the doctor the right to start a topic. Alternatively, the minimal *mmm* can also be heard to indicate the patient's understanding of the doctor's inquiry as being more interpersonal than instrumental and that the *mmm*-reception of the patient's information is an affiliative response to the doctor's interpersonal orientation. In either case, the doctor's further pursuit of social talk at line 8 indicates her orientation to relationship building at this point in the consultation, the accomplishment of which makes relevant core medical talk (line 10). Similar in its functions to the weather talk in Extract 6, talk related to the patient's work serves as a natural transition to the core instrumental frame of the consultation. The engagement in such talk could alleviate the patient's nervousness in seeking medical assistance and lessen the hierarchical distance between participants (Ragan, 2000).

```
(8) When did you arrive?
01  D: ni JIdianzhong dao       de  a?
       you when        arrive PRT PRT
       When did you arrive?
02     (.)
03  D: ↑liang ayi    a: ni SHENme shihou dao     de?
       Liang aunt PRT you what    when   arrive PRT
       ↑ Aunt Liang when did you arrive?
04  P: °( )dao          de°
            arrive PRT
       °I arrived at ( )°.
05  D: shenme SHIHOU] dao      de  yiyuan?
        what    when   arrive PRT hospital
       WHEN did you arrive at the hospital?
06     7.30 dao      de  ma?
       7.30 arrive PRT PRT
       At 7.30?
07  P: um
       mmm
       Mmm.
08  D: xianzai ganjue: zenme bu   hao?
       now         feel   how  not good
       how did you feel now? What's wrong?
```

When the patient sits down, the doctor greets her by asking when she arrives. Talk about the patient's time of arrival is certainly not related to the medical agenda of the current visit. Instead, it can be heard as being relational and interpersonal, indicating the doctor's care for the patient as a person who might have waited for a while before her current turn. When the doctor fails to receive an immediate response from the patient (line 2), she first addresses the patient in a heightened voice and then repeats her question. Here, by addressing the patient, the doctor displays her respect to the patient as a senior. In that sense, the doctor's addressing turn at line 3 is relational-oriented, dwarfing her professional identity and thereby shortening the hierarchical distance between herself and the patient. While the patient's information-giving is difficult to capture, given her extremely low voice (line 4), the doctor reiterates her inquiry (line 6). Immediately in her second TCU, the doctor makes an assumption and formulates her inquiry, making a simple yes/no-response relevant. It could be possible that the doctor is trying to reduce the difficulty of the question. It is also likely that by designing the question as a yes/no interrogative, the doctor indicates her orientation to close the topic and move to the next item on the agenda. As we can see, after the patient's confirmation of the doctor's assumption, the doctor announces a frame shift to the core medical agenda via a general inquiry, making patient presentation relevant.

The relational function of such talk is more pronounced in Extract (9) below. The doctor finds that the patient is down and tries to encourage her engagement in the conversation.

```
(9) Talk to me
01  D:  jintian zenme le   a::? YOU    bugaoxing le   a?
        today   what  PRT PRT  again unhappy    PRT PRT
        What happened today? you seem unhappy again?
02      kan shangqu haoxiang: jingshen bu   hao   me
        look PRT     as if         mood    not good PRT
        You seem to be in a bad mood today.
03      (0.2)
04      a?
        PRT
        A?
05      (0.4)
06  D:  hehe (.) zenme la?
        hheh      what  PRT
        Hhheh (.) what's up?
07      (0.5)
08  D:  ni ziji lai  de a?
        you own come PRT PRT
        you came here alone?
09      (0.2)
10  D:  A?  shi ni ziji lai   de ma?
        PRT is  you own come PRT PRT
        A? Did you come here alone?
11      jintian haoxiang bu duijing me?
        today   seem      not right  PRT
        She seems not right?
12  F:  MEIyou a
        no     PRT
        No.
```

```
13  D: meiyou a
        no       PRT
        No

14  D: hao   bu    hao a?
        good  not  good PRT
        Are you okay or not?

15     gen wo shuo liang ju        hua  lei
       to  me talk  two  sentence  talk PRT
       Talk to me *lei*.

16     hehehe
       Heh heh heh
       Heh heh heh

17     (0.5)

18     lai(.) shetou kan yixia
       come    tongue show PRT
       Come (.) show me your tongue.
```

The sequence opens with the doctor noticing the patient's unusual behavior. In line 1, the doctor's opening inquiry about what happened to the patient displays her care for the psychological or emotional status of the patient. The inquiry into the patient's emotive state (lines 1–2) conveys the doctor's care for the patient. Where the doctor's inquiry is non-reciprocated (line 3), the doctor first produces laughter (line 6). Here, the turn-initial laughter after the lapse functions as a remedy (Gavioli, 2009; Haakana, 2001), alleviating the potential awkwardness caused by the silence. Alternatively, the turn-initial *hehe* can also be heard as putting the patient at ease, making patient information-giving relevant. After a secondary lapse (line 7), the doctor announces a topic shift to a more neutral or uncontroversial topic, asking the patient if she came to the hospital alone (line 8). This inquiry is clearly phatic, as the patient's daughter is sitting next to her. In other words, the doctor's inquiry here is not produced for an answer. In her next turn at line 11, the doctor tries to find out what happened to the patient from her daughter. Therefore, the doctor is quite clear in understanding that the patient does not come alone. The function of the utterance is to encourage patient engagement in the current interaction. The propitiatory function of small talk is most salient at line 15, where the doctor asks the patient to talk to her. Again, the doctor's request lapses into silence (line 17). The three lapses can be fairly treated as 'conspicuous absence of talk' (Hoey, 2015, p. 442). One possible explanation, as the extract shows, is that the patient is not in a good mood to engage in small talk with the doctor. After repeated failure at invoking patient participation, the doctor announces a frame shift to the institutional agenda of the medical encounter by carrying out a physical examination of the patient. In the above extract, small talk is integrated into the core medical talk. While indicating care, intimacy, and friendliness, questions about the recipient's emotive status in medical encounters can invite patient presentation of their problems and troubles (Jefferson, 2015).

7.3.3 Administrative talk at medical openings

Prior research has agreed that small talk in various medical consultations involves some 'boundary-crossing activities' (Marra et al., 2017, p. 228). Hudak and Maynard (2011, p. 647) introduced the concept of 'co-topical small talk', which is usually interspersed between instrumental talk at certain points in the consultation. According to Hudak and Maynard, co-topical small talk is related to the ongoing medical agenda while other actions are taking place. They argue that activities such as bantering and complimenting, which invoke participants' institutional identities, should be considered as such. In the TCM corpora, there is another type of co-topical small talk – talk related to the administrative service, similar in its function to the *future arrangement sequence* (Schegloff & Sacks, 1973). While earlier studies suggested that such a sequence normally occurs in the closing phase of the consultation (West, 2006), it may also occur in medical openings. In Extract (10), the doctor advises the patient to book an appointment for the next visit and explained in detail the logistics.

```
(10) Go and book now
01  D: tamen dou shi XIAN      yuyue     de   haozi
       they  all are in advance reserve   PRT  number
       They make the reservation IN ADVANCE.
02  P: dui   de    dui de
       right PRT right PRT
       Right right.
03  F: wo xiaci      YE    wangshang gua
       i  next time also online     reserve
       Next time I will also make a reservation online.
04     ↑ wangshang keyi gua     de   ou?
         online     can reserve PRT PRT
       I can reserve online right?
05  P: MEISHI      meishi
       never mind never mind
       Never mind, never mind.
06     women xiaci      ye wangshang gua
       we    next time also online   reserve
       Next time, we will also make the reservation online.
07  D: jintian jiu   qu  yue
       today   just go reserve
       Make a reservation today.
08  P: jintian jiu   qu yuyue    a?
       today   just go reserve PRT
       Make a reservation today?
09  D: dao fuwutai ↑MASHANG
       to  information desk
       Go to the information desk ↑IMMEDIATELY,
```

```
10      qu yuyue     qu
        to reserve to
        and make a reservation.

11  P:  ou (.) wangshang meiyou gua     zhuanjia       de    ou?
        PRT    online    no    reserve specialist   PRT   PRT
        Ou (.) online reservation does not provide service
        for specialist care, right?

12  D:  zheyang KUAI (.)
        this    fast
        This is FAST (.)

13      ni dao wangshang dehua GENG Man
        you to online     if    more slow
        It will be even SLOWER if you book online.

14  P:  ou
        PRT
        Ou.

15  D:  youdeshihou hai rongyi man diao
        sometimes  will likely full PRT
        Sometimes it will be fully booked

16      [mei de   gua]
         no  PRT reserve
        [you cannot make the reservation]

17  P:  [wo shi jide     1.30 gua      de]
         I   am  remember 1.30 reserve PRT
        [I remember that I made the reservation at 1.30.]

18  D:  bu  yiding   de
        not necessary PRT
        Not necessarily.

19      [tamen youshihou shuobuding] yijing   yue  man le
         they  sometimes maybe       already book full PRT
        [Sometimes they might be] already fully booked.

20  P:  [bu   yiding   de a?]
         not necessary PRT PRT
        [Not necessarily?]

21      zheyang de    a
        this    PRT PRT
        That's how it is.

22  D:  ni haishi zhege: fuwutai          qu KANyikan
        you better this  information desk to see
        You'd better check at the information desk.

23  P:  ou
        PRT
        Ou.

24  D:  yaobu yihuier Wo zheli bang ni kanyikan
        or    later   I  here  help you see
        Or I can check it for you on my computer later.
```

```
25  (0.2)
26  D: shetou gei wo Kankan
       tongue to  me see
       Show me your tongue.
```

In this extract, the doctor advises the patient to make an appointment immediately at the appointment desk. Small talk in this extract takes the form of administrative talk. The doctor opens the conversation by providing the reasons for the patient's long wait (line 1), displaying a sense of friendliness and an orientation toward relationship building. The doctor's explanation can be heard as warding off any negative affect. As Dagger et al. (2007) note in a consumer context, timeliness is an important variable in explaining customers' perceptions of the administrative quality of a service encounter. In that sense, the administrative talk sequence in the medical setting serves a propitiatory function (Coupland et al., 1994). The patient contributes to the construction of small talk by showing understanding (lines 2–6). The consecutive articulation of 'never mind' at line 5 and the announcement of future activities at line 6 indicate the patient's orientation toward the long wait as being attributable to her failure to make an appointment online in advance rather than to the administrative quality of the service. In response to the patient's announcement, the doctor suggests the patient make an appointment in the here-and-now interaction (lines 7–10) and provides justifications for her advice (lines 12–19), making acceptance relevant. At line 23, the patient's use of the free-standing *ou*, similar in its function to *oh* in English (see Wu, 2004; Heritage, 1984), minimally receives the prior informing and could be sufficient to propose an acceptance, indicating a possible closing of the current topic. While the patient's *ou* makes a topic termination and topic shift relevant, the doctor pursues topic continuation by offering more assistance (line 24).

In most of my data, such an administrative talk sequence usually occur in medical closings as the last activity before the terminal exchange (Schegloff & Sacks, 1973). Extract 10 is an ad hoc case that illustrates the possibility of engaging in talk about future arrangement activities as the first interactional task in medical consultations. The doctor in the above interaction provides an excellent example of how talk, which is not strictly instrumental yet related to the ongoing medical agenda, functions to ward off any potential negative affect, thereby displaying the speaker's friendliness and building rapport.

7.4 Small talk at medical closings

In both TCM and WM consultations, small talk primarily occurs at the closing stage: in 90% of the TCM and 44% of the WM closings. A closer inspection of the texture of small talk suggests a clinical difference in the forms and sequences of small talk.

7.4.1 Social talk at medical closings

Laver (1975) noted that topics of small talk at the closing stage are mostly related to personal topics. He argued that non-controversial topics seldom occur in the closing stage. Findings of the present TCM data are at odds with Laver's observation: doctors and patients in TCM closings actively engage in social talk on various topics, both personal and non-controversial. Consider Extract 11, where discussions about the prescription invokes talk about the urban post service.

```
(11) Urban post service
01  D: ni   dai   jian   de   ou?
        you help concoct PRT PRT
        We concoct the herbal medicine for you, right?
02  P: ai
        yep
        Yep.
03  ((The doctor prepares the homeopathic prescription))
04  D: na   shi: youji gei ni shiba?
        then is   post  to you right
        By post, right?
05  P: ai youji
        yep post
        Yep, by post.
06  (0.4)
07  P: song song ye: MAN     lihai        de   ne
        post post too very large quantity PRT PRT
        A large quantity to deliver.
08  D: zhexie dou shi kuaidi        song   de
        these  all are post service deliver PRT
        These will be delivered by the post service.
09  P: kuaidi        song   de a?
        post service deliver PRT PRT
        By the post service?
10  D: shi de
        yes PRT
        Yes.
11  P: ou
        PRT
        Ou.
12     youyitian song   dao wo jia yijing  qidian duo   le
        once     deliver to  my home already 7     more PRT
           There was once when they arrived, it was more than 7.
13     shangyici SHIDIAN dou    mei dao
        last time 10      still  no at
        and last time when they arrived, it was not 10 yet.
```

```
14  D: ta shi: youzheng song      de haishi nage:-
       it is   postal   deliver PRT or    that
       Is it by the postal bureau or-?
15  P: ai< bushi youzheng
       yep not   postal
       Yep< no, not by the postal bureau.
16  ((The doctor hands over the homeopathic prescription))
17  D: hao
       okay
       Okay.
```

In the interaction above, talk about the urban post service (line 4 and thereafter) is invoked by participants' prior discussions about the patient's preference for an herbal compounding approach (lines 1–2). The doctor's prescription preparation at line 3 announces a frame shift to a closing-relevant environment (Schegloff & Sacks, 1973). At line 4, the doctor checks with the patient whether the herbal medicines would be sent to him by mail. In so asking, the doctor indicates her orientation toward the current interaction as being more interpersonal, where topics less related to the instrumental agenda are legitimately allowed. While the patient's *yes*-response (line 5) is sufficient to answer the doctor's question, it is not designed to invite or invoke further discussion, as evidenced by the silence at line 6. After the silence, the patient resumes the prior discussion by providing an evaluation of the mail service. By suggesting the heavy workload of the service, the patient designs his turn as gossip, making gossip relevant. Thereafter, an extensive gossip sequence emerges as a natural sequential next activity (lines 8–15). The sequence is closed by the doctor's handing him the prescription (line 16), indicating a sequence closure.

Given the sequential location – between the instrumental activities of preparing the prescription and handing the prescription to the patient – small talk in the above interaction primarily serves the function of silence filling (Benwell & McCreaddie, 2016; Jin, 2020; Maynard & Hudak, 2008). Alternatively, engagement in trivial and unserious topics constructs relationship building. However, it should be noted that it is the doctor who licenses the small talk in the here-and-now interaction. First, in line 4, the doctor's announcement of a frame shift indicates her orientation toward small talk as an appropriate activity in the interaction underway. Then, at line 16, the doctor suggests a sequence closure by handing over the prescription. In that sense, the doctor determines how much small talk is allowed in the ongoing interaction. The engagement in small talk foregrounds participants' social identities and mitigates the hierarchical difference between their institutional identities.

A similar sequence is illustrated in Extract 12. Small talk about the urban mail service is invoked by talk about the compounding arrangement.

```
(12) New address for herbal post
01  ((The doctor calls the next patient for preparation))
```

```
02  D: ziji jian     haishi dai jian?
       self concoct   or   help concot
       Will you concoct by yourself or leave it to us?
03  P: dai  jian  de
       help concoct PRT
       I will leave it to you.
04     (.)
05  P: wo MINGtian lai    na  ou
       I   tomorrow come take PRT
       I will collect it TOMOrrow.
06  D: song      de =mianfei song     de
       deliver PRT  free    deliver PRT
       By post =free delivery.
07  P: ou   hao de   hao de
       PRT okay PRT okay PRT
       Ou okay, okay.
08  (0.3)
09  P: xianzai shenme    dou keyi yong kuaidi
       now       anything all can  use   post
       Nowadays, everything can be delivered by post.
10  D: DUOshao fangbian     la
       how        convenient PRT
       HOw convenient.
11  P: ai: xianzai dou wangshang mai mai hao le
       yep now      all online     buy buy can PRT
       Ye:p now everything can be bought online,
12     gao ge nage zhifubao
       use PRT that Alipay
       by the use of Alipay.
13  ((The doctor hands over the homeopathic prescription))
14  P: ei: hao de    xiexie    yisheng ou
       PRT okay PRT thank you doctor    PRT
       Ei: okay, thank you doctor.
15  D: um
       mmm
       Mmm.
```

The doctor's calling the next patient to get ready announces a frame shift from the prior activity to the closing-relevant environment, making relevant some final activities, one of which is the arrangement of the patient's compounding preference. In line 7, the patient accepts the doctor's advice about having her herbal medicines delivered by mail. At this point, the activity of arranging for concoction is potentially complete. Here, both the doctor and the patient forego the option to speak, making relevant the emergence of a lapse at line 8. While a lapse at a transition-relevance place makes relevant various activities such as ending the interaction, starting a new topic, and continuing the current topic (Hoey, 2018), the patient opts to start a new topic using materials from the prelapse sequence. The doctor's responsive turn at line 10 ratifies the patient's proposal and co-constructs the small-talk sequence. Thus far, both the doctor and the patient have displayed an orientation toward the ongoing interaction as silence filling and relationship building. The small-talk sequence terminates at line 13 with the doctor's handing over the prescription. Here, the doctor's action can be heard as a pre-closing (Schegloff & Sacks, 1973). The patient aligns with the doctor and co-constructs the closing by providing the canonical thank-you formula (line 14).

Talk about personal topics also occurred in TCM closings. In Extract 13, the discussion on the patient's psychological wellness can be considered as co-topical. Such talk later develops into some topicalized small talk (Hudak & Maynard, 2011).

```
(13) Being a boss
01 ********** ((The printing machine is working))
02 D: ni yao laoban zuo  de   DA    yidian
       you if boss   work PRT larger a little
       If you run a larger business,
03     ni  jiu  xintai HEN  hao  le
       you will mindset very good PRT
       you will have a very positive mindset.
04 P: um
      mmm
      Mmm.
05 D: ni fanzheng: YIZHI xiang zuo  ge   da    laoban
      you anyway   always want work PRT  large boss
      Anyway you've ALWAYS wanted to run a large business.
06 P: zuo    da laoban ye   MEI na:me hao   zuo   a
      work large boss  also not  that easy work PRT
      It's NOT that easy to run a large business as we:ll.
07 D: hehe
      Hheh hheh
      Heheh.
08 P: zuo  da   laoban DOU shi maobing
      work large boss  all are illness
      People who have large businesses also have MULTIPLE illnesses.
09     women naxie laoban dou shi maobing
       our   those boss   all are illnesses
       Our bosses all full of illnesses.
10 ((The doctor signs the prescription))
11 D: aiya: keyi xiaban          le
      aiya  can  get off work PRT
      Aiya: time to get off work.
```

```
12  P:  heihei  (.)
        hheheh
        Hhehheh.

13      xiawu     ne? xiawu       bingfang?
        afternoon PRT afternoon   ward
        How about afternoon? In the ward?

14  D:  um
        mmm
        Mmm.

15      hao  le
        okay PRT
        Okay.

16  P:  um   xiexie    ou
        mmm  thank you PRT
        Mmm thank you.

17  D:  um   zou      hao
        mmm  goodbye  safe
        Mmm, bye and safe.
```

The printer printing the prescription suggests a shift to the closing-relevant environment. The doctor's indirect advice on keeping a positive mindset is a reinvocation of material talked about earlier in the conversation (Schegloff & Sacks, 1973). The advice thus nicely relates the patient's problem (insomnia) to his psychological well-being, making patient acceptance relevant. Here, the doctor formulates her advice in a way that is heard as being evaluative rather than persuasive. 'If you run a larger business, you will have a very positive mindset.' In so claiming, the doctor relates the patient's poor mentality to the size of his business rather than the patient himself. The doctor's turn here invokes the patient's identities as a boss and as a patient seeking medical assistance. In that sense, the doctor's turn can be considered as being co-topical. In response to the doctor's advice, the patient produces a minimal token indicating information receiving (line 4). From this point and onward, talk between the doctor and the patient develop into some sort of topicalized small talk, which is 'referentially independent from the institutional identities of the participants' (Hudak & Maynard, 2011, p. 647). The doctor's articulation of the patient's ambition at line 5 is occasioned by her prior advice. This topic is immediately picked up by the patient and later develops into a troubles-telling sequence (Jefferson, 2015). The patient does not align with the doctor's claim but instead suggests difficulty in running a large business (lines 6–9). The troubles-telling sequence is disattended to by the doctor, preventing it from becoming too big (see Benwell & McCreaddie, 2016). Instead, the doctor announces a possible pre-closing (line 11). In response to the doctor's announcement, the patient takes the opportunity to build the relationship by showing care to the doctor (lines 12–13). The visit ended shortly after the doctor announces a secondary pre-closing (line 15) and the patient expresses appreciation for the doctor's service (line 16). Like other forms of small talk, talk about personal matters in medical closings fills a gap between planned activities: the writing of the prescription and the closing of the consultation.

```
(14) Plans for the weekend
01  ******** ((Sound of the printer))
02  D: nimen zhege libai    BU guoqu a?
       you   this weekend not go    PRT
       You're not going there this weekend?
03  P: DUI (.) zhege libai    bu guoqu
       right    this  weekend not go
       No (.) not this weekend.
04  D: um
       mmm
       Mmm.
05  F: (            )
06  D: ou
       PRT
       Ou.
07  (0.8)
08  D: HEN  MAN  lei (.) yao deng    yixia
       very slow PRT     need wait a while
       It's VERY SLOW (.) you need to wait for a while.
09     xiayige xian
       next    first
       Who's next?
10  ((The doctor calls the next patient for preparation))
11  (5.8)
12  ((The doctor signs the homeopathic prescription))
13  D: nao
       here
       Here you are.
14  P: ou (.) xiexie    ou
       PRT    thank you PRT
       Ou(.) thank you.
```

In line 1, the doctor's printing the prescription marks a transition to the closing stage of the encounter. The doctor's question about how the patient will spend her weekends indicates her orientation toward the current interaction as relationship building, where talk involving issues less relevant to the core medical agenda is appropriate to emerge. The sequential position of the doctor's turn suggests that social talk in the above sequence functions as a time filler (Holmes, 2000). This expansion into social topics quickly develops within the conversation a sense of intimacy and friendliness (Coupland et al., 1994). In the presence of the third party, the doctor uses the plural *you*, thereby inviting both the patient and the family into the social talk. This orientation is immediately picked up by the family: in line 5, the husband extends the patient's response by providing reasons for their plan. Thus far, the doctor, the patient, and the family have collaboratively projected the relevance of social talk as the next activity of preparing the prescription in the closing-relevant environment. The doctor receives the husband's explanation with minimal acknowledgement, bringing the sequence into a possible completion where a lapse naturally occurred as the next action (line 7). At line 8, the doctor resolves the lapse by 'registering some perceptible aspect of the situated environment' (Hoey, 2018, p. 339). 'It's VERY SLOW (.) you need to wait for a while.' In so articulating, the doctor not only provides an explanation for not closing the encounter in the here-and-now interaction but also announces a termination of the prior social talk sequence. One possible underlying assumption of the doctor's statement is that upon the completion of the printing, the consultation shall come to an end. Another likely assumption is that the doctor has no particulars to mention at this stage, making ground for allowing her to call the next patient (line 9). It is thus sound to conclude that the social talk here functions as a silence avoidance strategy (Jaworski, 2000).

7.4.2 Thanking formulae

Common between WM and TCM closings is the observation of the thanking formulae as the terminal exchange (Schegloff & Sacks, 1973; West, 2006), constituting a phatic parting sequence. In several observations, such a parting sequence is unilateral.

```
(15)
01  D:  haole
        okay
        Okay.
02  P:  xiexie
        thank you
        Thank you.
03  D:  you    wenti   zai   lai   hao le
        have problem again come can PRT
        In case of other problems, come here again.
04  P:  ou   ou   xiexie
        PRT PRT thank you
        Ou ou thank you.

(16)
01  D:  zhege yao   shi zuo  changjing    de
        this  pill is  take colonoscopy PRT
        The pill is for the colonoscopy.
```

```
02  P: um    um wo zhidao
       mmm mmm I know
       Mmm mmm, I know.
03  D: ou
       PRT
       Ou.
04  P: xiexie
       thank you
       Thank you.
```

```
(17)
01  ((The doctor calls the next patient))
02  P: xieixe    yisheng
       thank you doctor
       Thank you, doctor.
```

```
(18)
01  D: nao ((hands over the homeopathic prescription))
       here
       Here you are.
02  P: xiexie    yisheng ou
       thank you doctor   PRT
       Thank you, doctor.
```

```
(19)
01  D: hao
       okay
       Okay.
02  P: xiexie    yisheng
       thank you doctor
       Thank you, doctor.
```

Extracts (15)–(17) are taken from WM consultations, and (18) and (19) are from TCM. In all these five extracts, the thanking formulae are produced after the doctor's possible pre-closing announcement and function as the terminal exchange. While the patient normally expresses their appreciation for the doctor's service, the doctor seldom responds making the thanking formulae unilateral. Moreover, when delivering their expression of gratitude, the patient normally addresses the doctor to convey their deference. It is likely that the doctor needs to attend to the next patient and has no time to respond to the current patient's leaving. In any case, the fact that most of the thanking is not responded to by the doctor points to the hierarchical difference in medical consultations.

In rare instances in TCM encounters, the doctor co-constructs the parting with the patient. Consider Extracts 20 and 21 below.

(20)
```
01  D: XING xiaci      zai     lai kankan ba
       fine next time again come see   PRT
       FINE come and see me next time.

02     ni   zhe  shou TAI zi    le
       you  this hand too purple PRT
       Your hands look TOO purple.

03  P: xing xiaci     zai    lai
       fine next time again  come
       Fine, come again next time.

04  D: ai: hao   lei =hao zaijian
       yep okay  PRT okay bye
       Ye:p okay =okay, bye.

05  P: xiexie     yisheng
       thank you  doctor
       Thank you, doctor.

06  D: ai
       yep
       Yep.
```

(21)
```
01  D: um
       mmm
       Mmm.

02     hao  le
       okay PRT
       Okay.

03  P: um   xiexie   ou
       mmm thank you PRT
       Mmm thank you.

04  D: um   zou      hao
       mmm goodbye safe
       Mmm, bye and safe.
```

While the rarity of the doctor's exchange of farewell or thanking in the parting sequence indicates a power asymmetry, it also points to some mutually accepted practices in both TCM and WM consultations regarding the patient's leaving.

7.5 Summary

The opening and closing stages of medical consultations constitute the boundaries of interaction, where relational work is usually involved, making relevant nonmedical small talk. Using a context-based approach to examine small talk, this chapter addresses where and how small talk emerges in TCM and WM encounters. The chapter also discusses the various functions small talk serves in different sequential placements. The three primary functions are silence filling, relationship building, and lubricating the transition to the core instrumental frame. Notwithstanding the importance of small talk in delivering patient-centered care, this chapter reports a rarity of small talk in medical consultations, particularly in WM encounters. The scarcity of small talk in WM thus reflects a conventional instrumental style of medical consultation. This chapter also introduces a new type of small talk: co-topical small talk, which features a duality in its relevance to the instrumental and interpersonal/social/relational agenda of the medical encounter. I have illustrated how co-topical small talk might include medically relevant information while attending to interpersonal goals.

The next chapter summarizes the major findings of the three independent studies and discusses the implications for both linguists and health practitioners.

References

Beck, C. S., & Ragan, S. L. (1992). Negotiating interpersonal and medical talk: Frame shifts in the gynecologic exam. *Journal of Language and Social Psychology, 11*(1–2), 47–61. https://doi.org/10.1177%2F0261927X92111004

Benwell, B., & McCreaddie, M. (2016). Keeping 'small talk' small in healthcare encounters: Negotiating the boundaries between on- and off-task talk. *Research on Language and Social Interaction, 49*(3), 258–271. https://doi.org/10.1080/08351813.2016.1196548

Coupland, J. (2000). Introduction: Sociolinguistic perspectives on small talk. In J. Coupland (Ed.), *Small talk* (pp. 1–25). Pearson Education. http://dx.doi.org/10.4324/9781315838328-1

Coupland, J., Coupland, N., & Robinson, J. D. (1992). 'How are you?': Negotiating phatic communion. *Language in Society, 21*(2), 207–230. https://doi.org/10.1017/S0047404500015268

Coupland, J., Robinson, J. D., & Coupland, N. (1994). Frame negotiation in doctor-elderly patient consultations. *Discourse and Society, 5*(1), 89–124. https://doi.org/10.1177%2F0957926594005001005

Dagger, T. S., Sweeney, J. C., & Johnson, L. W. (2007). A hierarchical model of health service quality. *Journal of Service Research, 10*(2), 123–142. https://doi.org/10.1177%2F1094670507309594

Defibaugh, S. (2018). Small talk as work talk: Enacting the patient-centered approach in nurse-practitioner-patient visits. *Communication & Medicine, 14*(2), 97–107. https://doi.org/10.1558/cam.31374

Fawole, A. A., & Rammala, J. R. (2021). Rapport management in the opening sequence of African and Asian doctors in South Africa. *International Journal of Applied Linguistics, 31*(3), 402–420. https://doi.org/10.1111/ijal.12338

Gardner, R. (2001). *When listeners talk: Response tokens and listener stance*. Amsterdam and Philadelphia: John Benjamins. https://doi.org/10.1075/pbns.92

Gavioli, L. (2009). Turn-initial versus turn-final laughter: Two techniques for initiating remedy in English/Italian bookshop service encounters. *Discourse Processes, 19*(3), 369–384. https://doi.org/10.1080/01638539509544923

Haakana, M. (2001). Laughter as a patient's resource: Dealing with delicate aspects of medical interaction. *Text & Talk, 21*(1–2), 187–219. https://doi.org/10.1515/text.1.21.1-2.187

Heritage, J. (1984). A change-of-state token and aspects of its sequential placement. In J. M. Atkinson & J. Heritage (Eds.), *Structures of social action: Studies in conversation analysis* (pp. 299–345). Cambridge: Cambridge University Press. https://doi.org/10.1017/CBO9780511665868.020

Heritage, J., & Robinson, J. D. (2006). The structure of patients' presenting concerns: Physicians' opening questions. *Health Communication, 19*(2), 89–102. https://doi.org/10.1207/s15327027hc1902_1

Hoey, E. M. (2015). Lapses: How people arrive at, and deal with, discontinuities in talk. *Research on Language and Social Interaction, 48*(4), 430–453. https://doi.org/10.1080/08351813.2015.1090116

Hoey, E. M. (2018). How speakers continue with talk after a lapse in conversation. *Research on Language and Social Interaction, 51*(3), 329–346. https://doi.org/10.1080/08351813.2018.1485234

Holmes, J. (2000). Doing collegiality and keeping control at work: Small talk in government departments. In J. Coupland (Ed.), *Small talk* (pp. 32–61). London: Pearson Education. https://doi.org/10.4324/9781315838328-3

Holmes, J. (2005). When small talk is a big deal: sociolinguistic challenges in the workplace. In M. H. Long (Ed.), *Second language needs analysis* (pp. 344–371). Cambridge: Cambridge University Press. https://doi.org/10.1017/CBO9780511667299.012

Holmes, J., & Stubbe, M. (2015). *Power and politeness in the workplace: A sociolinguistic analysis of talk at work* (2nd ed). London: Routledge. https://doi.org/10.4324/9781315750231

Holmes, J., & Woodhams, J. (2013). Building interaction: The role of talk in joining a community of practice. *Discourse & Communication, 7*(3), 275–298. https://doi.org/10.1177%2F1750481313494500

Holt, E. (2010). The last laugh: Shared laughter and topic termination. *Journal of Pragmatics, 42*(6), 1513–1525. https://doi.org/10.1016/j.pragma.2010.01.011

Hössjer, A. (2013). Small talk, politeness, and email communication in the workplace. In S. Herring, D. Stein, & T. Virtanen (Eds.), *Pragmatics of computer-mediated communication* (pp. 613–638). Berlin: Walter De Gruyter. https://doi.org/10.1515/9783110214468.613

Hudak, P. L., & Maynard, D. W. (2011). An interactional approach to conceptualizing small talk in medical interactions. *Sociology of Health & Illness, 33*(4), 634–653. https://doi.org/10.1111/j.1467-9566.2011.01343.x

Jaworski, A. (2000). Silence and small talk. In J. Coupland (Eds.), *Small talk* (pp. 110–132). London: Pearson Education. https://doi.org/10.4324/9781315838328-6

Jefferson, G. (2015). *Talking about troubles in conversation*. New York: Oxford University Press.

Jefferson, G., Sacks, H., & Schegloff, E. A. (1987). Notes on laughter in the pursuit of intimacy. In G. Button & J. R. E. Lee (Eds.), *Talk and social organization* (pp. 152–205). Clevedon: Multilingual Matters.

Jin, Y. (2020). Framing boundaries of medical interactions: Data from China. In B. Watson & J. Krieger (Eds.), *Expanding horizons in health communication: An Asian perspective* (pp. 107–131). Singapore: Springer Nature Singapore. https://doi.org/10.1007/978-981-15-4389-0_6

Laver, J. (1975). Communicative functions of phatic communion. In A. Kendon, R. M. Harris, & M. R. Key (Eds.), *Organization of behavior in face-to-face interaction* (pp. 215–238). The Hague and Paris: Mouton de Gruyter. https://doi.org/10.1515/9783110907643.215

Laver, J. (1981). Linguistic routines and politeness in greeting and parting. In F. Coulmas (Ed.), *Conversational routine: Explorations in standardized communication situations and prepatterned speech* (pp. 289–304). The Hague and Paris: Mouton. https://doi. org/10.1515/9783110809145.289

Mak, B. C. N. (2019). Doing business and constructing identities through small talk in workplace instant messaging. *Pragmatics and Society, 10*(4), 559–583. https://doi. org/10.1075/ps.16064.mak

Malinowski, B. (1923). The problem of meaning in primitive languages. In C. K. Ogden & I. A. Richards (Eds.), *The meaning of meaning* (pp. 296–336). London: Routledge & Kegan Paul.

Malinowski, B. (1972). The problem of meaning in primitive languages. In C. K. Ogden & I. A. Richards (Eds.), *The meaning of meaning* (10th ed., pp. 296–336). New York: Routledge & Kegan Paul.

Marra, M., Holmes, J., & Kidner, K. (2017). Transitions and interactional competence: Negotiating boundaries through talk. In S. P. Doehler, A. Bangerter, G. de Weck, L. Filliettaz, E. González-Martínez, & C. Petitjean (Eds.), *Interactional competences in institutional settings: From school to the workplace* (pp. 227–251). Cham, Switzerland: Palgrave Macmillan. https://doi.org/10.1007/978-3-319-46867-9_9

Maynard, D. W., & Hudak, P. L. (2008). Small talk, high stakes: Interactional disattentiveness in the context of prosocial doctor–patient interaction. *Language in Society, 37*(5), 661–688. https://doi.org/10.1017/S0047404508080986

Penn, C., & Watermeyer, J. (2012). When asides become central: Small talk and big talk in interpreted health interactions. *Patient Education and Counseling, 88*(3), 391–398. https://doi.org/10.1016/j.pec.2012.06.016

Pomerantz, A. (1980). Telling my side: 'Limited access' as a 'fishing' device. *Sociological Inquiry, 50*(3–4), 186–198. https://doi.org/10.1111/j.1475-682X.1980.tb0 0020.x

Ragan, S. L. (2000). Sociable talk in women's health care contexts: Two forms of non-medical talk. In J. Coupland (Ed.), *Small talk* (pp. 269–287). London: Pearson Education. http://dx.doi.org/10.4324/9781315838328-15

Raymond, G. (2003). Grammar and social organization: Yes/no interrogatives and the structure of responding. *American Sociological Review, 68*(6), 939–967. https:// psycnet.apa.org/doi/10.2307/1519752

Roberts, C. (2008). Intercultural communication in healthcare settings. In H. Kotthoff & H. Spencer-Oatey (Eds.), *Handbook of intercultural communication* (pp. 243–262). Berlin: Mouton De Gruyter. https://doi.org/10.1515/9783110198584.3.243

Roberts, C., & Sarangi, S. (1999). Hybridity in gatekeeping discourse: Issues of practical relevance for the researcher. In S. Sarangi & C. Roberts (Eds), *Talk, work and institutional order: Discourse in medical, mediation and management settings* (pp. 473–503). Berlin: Mouton De Gruyter. https://doi.org/10.1515/97831102 08375.4.473

Robinson, J. D. (1998). Getting down to business: Talk, gaze, and body orientation during openings of doctor–patient consultations. *Human Communication Research, 25*(1), 97–123. https://doi.org/10.1111/j.1468-2958.1998.tb00438.x

Schegloff, E. A., & Sacks, H. (1973). Opening up closings. *Semiotica, 8,* 289–327. https://doi.org/10.1515/semi.1973.8.4.289

Schneider, K. P. (1988). *Small talk: Analyzing phatic discourse.* Marburg: Hitzeroth.

Stivers, T. (2004). 'No no no' and other types of multiple sayings in social interaction. *Human Communication Research, 30*(2), 260–293. https://doi.org/10.1111/ j.1468-2958.2004.tb00733.x

Van der Laaken, M., & Bannink, A. (2020). Openings in follow-up cancer consultations: The 'How are you?' question revisited. *Discourse Studies, 22*(2), 205–220. https://doi.org/10.1177%2F1461445619893793

West, C. (2006). Coordinating closings in primary care visits: Producing continuity of care. In J. Heritage & D. W. Maynard (Eds.), *Communication in medical care: Interaction between primary care physicians and patients* (pp. 379–415). Cambridge: Cambridge University Press. https://doi.org/10.1017/CBO9780511607172.015

Wu, R-J. R. (2004). *Stance in talk: A conversation analysis of Mandarin final particles.* Amsterdam: John Benjamins. https://doi.org/10.1075/pbns.117

8 Summary, implications, and future directions

8.1 Introduction

In the preceding chapters, I have combined process analysis with Conversation Analysis to explore the similarities and differences between TCM and WM in relation to doctor–patient communication. The research is designed to contribute to the fields of health communication and discourse analysis by conducting an empirical study in two types of medical practices, with a particular focus on the activity types collaboratively accomplished by participants. The research is conversation-analytic in orientation and presents real-life interactions in chronic care to capture the social dynamic within which medicine is practiced.

With this in mind, I begin this concluding chapter by revisiting the research design and objectives. Then I go on to offer a synthesized summary of the findings in the three methodologically independent studies. Chapters 3 to 7 have been concerned with exploring the clinical similarities and differences in relation to doctor–patient communication behaviors and patient satisfaction. In the final part of this chapter, I highlight the implications and future directions of the findings for both communication and discourse researchers and health practitioners.

8.2 Revisiting the research design and objectives

The thrust of this research can be summarized as follows:

1. Given the high mortality rates caused by chronic diseases worldwide (WHO, 2003) and their strong age-dependent relation (Prince et al., 2015), communication in routine encounters where such diseases are monitored is subject to comprehensive analysis. An investigation invoking interactional approaches enriches our understanding of *what* is happening and *how* it happens as such in talk in situ.
2. The recent inclusion of TCM in WHO's global medical compendium (Cyranoski, 2018) indicates an increasing recognition of TCM as an alternative approach to WM in providing healthcare. Yet, the two medical practices have their own ways of treating the patient. A contextual analysis can

DOI: 10.4324/9781003161929-8

differentiate one medical practice from another and inform the institutional dynamic within which medicine is practiced.

Using an integration of qualitative and quantitative methods, this research extends prior research by uncovering the communication behaviors between doctors and patients in both TCM and WM practiced in China. The chapters in the book are organized to build conversation-analytic studies of specific activity types upon quantitative analyses of general communication patterns. By doing this, the book streamlines the macro findings (the big pictures of doctor–patient communication and patient satisfaction) with a top-down approach. On another level, the application of CA to specific activity types presents a bottom-up investigation on the structures of social actions (Atkinson & Heritage, 1984) and the ways through which participants collaboratively accomplish specific interactional tasks by relying on various linguistic resources. In other words, this research assigns priority to the qualitative part of the analyses. The combination of various methods in this sequence optimizes the effectiveness of a CA-driven study, focusing on what participants do and how they do it in situated contexts.

8.3 A synthesized summary of the findings

The process analysis and the microanalysis presented in Chapters 3–7 provide empirical evidence of the clinical similarities and differences in how doctors and patients engage in medical interactions in routine encounters. These findings can be summarized with the following statements:

(1) TCM and WM have different approaches for diagnosis and treatment, which affects the communication practice in medical encounters.

Findings of the preceding chapters have shown that TCM and WM doctors assign priority to different activities in medical consultations. The biggest difference lies in communication involving lifestyles, diagnostic testing, and nonmedical small talk. Through a closer examination of the sequential environments of these activities and the interactional work they accomplished, this study has shown that these activities are well organized for institutional goals.

With respect to lifestyle discussions, this study has focused on two activities: advice-giving and reception in TCM encounters. I noted that lifestyle advice regularly emerges in response to the formulation of a problem, suggesting a connection between the patient's problem and their lifestyle habits. In so presenting the advice, the doctor indicates the patient's behaviors as a possible cause of the problem, making acceptance relevant. Lifestyle advice may also emerge comfortably after a diagnostic statement, functioning as a treatment option. A unique place where lifestyle advice occurs in TCM consultations is the closing-relevant environment. Its emergence commonly functions as a take-home note and invites the patient to the reading that this is the last activity in the consultation. It may be used as a reminder of a behavioral change, or to promote health. In either case, the (re)introduction of lifestyle-related topics in the closing stage of the consultation displays the doctor's care to the patient.

In WM consultations, the diagnosis and treatment of a problem are mostly based on diagnostic testing. I have focused on the activity of diagnostic recommendation, which, according to the survey findings, is dominant in WM dialogues. The place where a diagnostic test recommendation frequently emerges is after the patient's problem presentation. Notably, this activity occurs even before the doctor's inquiry about the patient's medical history. The recommendation is to invite the patient to the reading that nothing is more reliable than diagnostic testing to understand their condition. It can preempt other activities at this stage of the interaction: by foregrounding diagnostic testing among other activities in an environment where information collection is underway, the doctor disattends to question-asking and postpones diagnosis. As patients reported, WM dialogues are full of diagnostic testing recommendations, with few questions about the patient's condition. The recommendation may also occur after the patient's orientation toward the relevance of diagnostic testing. When placed in this position, the recommendation emerges naturally and comfortably as an alignment to the patient's orientation. One particular observation in WM consultation is the doctor's announcement of a temporary closing or interruption of the current interaction. The doctor may require the patient to come and see her later with a diagnostic test report. The amount of time it takes to get the results depends on the type of test. In that sense, the diagnosis and subsequent treatment are postponed.

The paramountcy of diagnostic testing in WM might also account for the doctor's less attentive listening to the patient's story. As a critical part of the delivery of healthcare in WM, diagnostic testing is widely used to identify the cause of symptoms or diseases. Compared with patient narration, it is a more scientific way to understand the patient's condition. This is not to deny the importance of patient narration in WM consultations. Rather, WM places more weight on diagnostic testing than patient narration in understanding the patient's condition. By contrast, listening to patient narration is one of the key skills required in TCM diagnosis. Before WM was introduced into China, TCM diagnosis was heavily dependent on the four steps of inspection, auscultation and olfaction, inquiry, and palpation. In that sense, patients were and still are regarded as experts on their own health.

The differences in doctors' treatment of lifestyles and diagnostic testing could be attributed to the various diagnostic and therapeutic approaches in TCM and WM. TCM emphasizes holism and takes this approach when treating the patient, making relevant talk that invokes the patient's lifeworlds. In contrast, WM is evidence-based medicine, which places more weight on molecular and cellular changes when explaining diseases. This difference is reflected in the communication practice. Such difference could also explain the rarity of small talk in WM, not just in the form of phatic communion. The scarcity of small talk in WM conversations seems to reflect the participants' priority on insisting on the biomedical agenda of the encounter by focusing on the 'voice of medicine'

(Mishler, 1984). Alternatively, the preponderance of diagnostic tests with those daunting indices that seem to be esoteric to the doctor can intimidate the patient from engaging in interpersonal tasks. In contrast, with more reliance on patient narration and less reliance on diagnostic testing, TCM consultations are more relaxed and less instrumental.

(2) Medical consultations in routine encounters are instrumental and task-oriented. This is particularly the case in WM encounters.

Previous research on acute encounters has generally agreed that medical consultations are task-oriented, with the dominance of doctor-initiated questions and talk invoking instrumental tasks. A similar observation is found in routine encounters.

First, medical consultations in the present corpora usually open without small talk of any kind. Instead, conversations start with either the patient's formulation of a problem or the doctor's question eliciting patient concerns. This is particularly the case in WM consultations. The lack of transition to the core medical agenda at the opening phase suggests that medical consultations are strictly goal-directed (Gu, 1996). In addition, a closer examination of the sequential environments of small talk shows that it primarily serves to fill the silence between instrumental tasks, particularly at the closing phase of the encounter. In other words, rather than interrupting (Benwell & McCreaddie, 2016) or disattending instrumental tasks (Maynard & Hudak, 2008), small talk primarily functions to naturally transition to an interrupted or the next instrumental activity while other interpersonal tasks are simultaneously performed.

Second, the consultations observed in the present corpora are strikingly shorter than those reported in the literature (Deveugele et al., 2002; Geraghty et al., 2007; Irving et al., 2017; Wilson & Childs, 2002). Several studies have indicated an association between the content and the length of the consultation (Gude et al., 2013; Howie et al., 1991). As Deveugele et al. (2002) proposed, consultations in which psychosocial issues were considered important usually last longer than those with more emphasis on solving biomedical problems. This could possibly explain why WM consultations are noticeably shorter than TCM consultations in the present corpora, given the larger number of discussions about diagnostic testing rather than the patient's lifeworlds. Scholars have also related the length of consultation to the extent of patient-centeredness (Howie et al., 1992; Orton & Gray, 2016). As Taylor (2009) claimed, the duration of consultation has some bearing on the degree of patient-centeredness and patient satisfaction. Therefore, in the current research, patients are more satisfied with TCM doctors than WM doctors. Yet, the short consultation time should be read with caution. Prior research has suggested that most of the doctors in China's tertiary hospitals are overworked (Fu et al., 2018; Tu et al., 2015). According to the National Health and Family Planning Commission of China, there were 2.3 billion outpatient visits to Chinese hospitals, 46% of which were received by tertiary hospitals (Hu & Zhang, 2015; Tang et al., 2019). According to the 2014 National Survey, 92% of doctors in tertiary hospitals need to work overtime, and on average, 72% work more than 60 hours per week (Hu & Zhang, 2015), far beyond the legal limit of 44 hours (Fu et al., 2018). Therefore, the limited consultation time could be a trade-off for the heavy patient loads.

Finally, in my observation, most patients visit their doctors for at least one of the three purposes: to present a new symptom related to their chronic condition, to monitor their chronic condition (e.g., regular check-ups), and to obtain a medication refill. In the first two cases, doctors might request that the patient provide sufficient information to shown an understanding of their condition: in TCM, this is primarily accomplished through question-asking, whereas in WM, such information is derived mainly from diagnostic testing. Therefore, as we can find in the RIAS study (Figure 3.1), TCM doctors asked significantly more questions than WM doctors did in medical consultations ($p < 0.01$). When the patient's primary concern is to have their medication refilled, consultations are usually shorter than those in the first two cases. In TCM, the medicinal formula is specifically designed according to the patient and the consultation. In other words, refill of the same homeopathic prescription is less likely. The doctor writes the formula each time, with some modifications of the type or the dosage of the herbs. This process is impossible to complete without a close examination of the patient. On the other hand, the refill of medications in WM encounters can be accomplished within short exchanges, as in Extracts (1) and (2) below.

```
(1) Nexium refill
01  P: yisheng wo jiushi pei     nage:: nage: naixin
        doctor   I  just   refill that       that Nexium
        Doctor I just want to refill tha::t tha:t nexium.
02  D: ni   naixin GANG pei   guo de  ai
        you Nexium just refill have PRT PRT
        You HAVE just had the Nexium refilled.
((lines omitted))
09  P: na     xiaci   wo jiu   suan    hao
        then next time I just calculate PRT
        Then next time, I just need to wait
10      shijian bangeyue
        time      half a month
        for half a month.
11  D: (   ) hai  yao   ma?   [jiu pannixilin?]
             still want PRT     just Penicillin
        Do you still want ( )? [Just penicillin?]
12  P:                       [jiu: yiyang      ] ai
                              just    same        yep
                              [Just the same] yep
13  (3.5)
```

```
14  P:  na   wo jiu  15 hao  lai  hao  le  ou?
        then I  just  15 date come fine PRT PRT
        Then I just come on the 15th?

15  D:  yao  bangeyue
        need half a month
        In half a month.

16  P:  bangeyue yihou ai
        half a month    yep
        Half a month, yep.

17  D:  hao  le
        okay PRT

18  P:  haode xiexie
        okay  thank you
        Okay, thank you.
```

The interaction above is goal-oriented. The sequence starts with the patient's request for a medication refill, establishing her reason for the current visit, and making acceptance/rejection relevant. In addition, the articulation of a specific medication displays the patient's knowledge about his condition and foreshadows the forthcoming interaction as a service encounter where the patient is the consumer and the doctor is the provider (see Roter et al., 1997 for the consumerist encounter). The patient's request is challenged by the doctor, based on the time duration between her current medication refill and her last visit being too short. The hospital has a medication refill policy with strict requirements on the time allowed for the next refill. In response to the doctor's challenge, which can be heard as a rejection of the request, the patient produces extensive explanations with a further request on medication refill (lines 3–10, data not shown), which is accepted by the doctor. The doctor's alignment with the patient's orientation toward the ongoing interaction as a consumerist encounter is evidenced at line 11: by asking the patient if he needed other medications, the doctor proffers the patient the right to make the medication decisions. Upon the doctor's fulfillment of the patient's request, the conversation closes with the patient's showing of gratitude, displaying his satisfaction with the doctor's service. Such a sequence is more evident in Extract 2.

```
(2) Statins refill
01  P:  peiyao
        medication refill
        Medication refill.

02  D:  um
        mmm
        Mmm.

03  P:  na:ge zhongliu pian haiyou tating
        that  tumor  pill and    statins
        Tha:t tumor pill and statins.
```

```
04  D: tating    a?
       statins PRT
       Statins?
05  P: DUI     tating  ,
       right statins
       Right statins.
06  D: nazhong tating?
       which     statins
       Which one?
((lines omitted))
32  D: um    hao  le
       mmm  okay  PRT
       Mmm okay.
```

The patient opens the consultation with a short and straightforward announce-ment of her reason for the current visit (line 1). The patient's naming of the medicine (line 3) indicates her knowledge about the medicine, including its ingredients, functions, directions, and cautions. In other words, rather than being a layperson, the patient builds her identity as a knowledgeable person. The doctor aligns with the patient's orientation by asking the patient to specify the type of the drug (line 6). The sequence presented here is similar to that in other service encounters such as a café, where the waitress asks the customer which specific coffee they want. Thereafter, the patient and the doctor work together toward a medication refill (lines omitted). In both Extracts, the patient is the active client while the doctor is a passive provider. Such a sequence is absent in TCM encounters.

8.4 Implications and future directions

Finally, I wish to offer some future directions by suggesting other approaches to medical discourse and communication research. These suggestions are intended to build upon the present findings.

8.4.1 Implications for communication and discourse scholars and health practitioners

This research combines top-down and bottom-up approaches to examine doctor–patient communication and patient satisfaction between two medical practices in China. To my knowledge, this is one of the few studies that compare two medical practices with various philosophies and diagnostic approaches. Given the trend of using TCM in various healthcare encounters (e.g., treatment of cancer and COVID-19), understanding the differences is necessary for professional-client and intra-professional communication.

Three methodologically independent studies are included. The RIAS study provides a summarization of the activities observed in medical encounters. To my knowledge, this is the first study to apply RIAS to TCM consultations. Therefore, the findings derived from the RIAS study have practical implications for informing clinical practice and patient expectations and decisions for medical care in China and elsewhere, where the two clinical practices coexist. The study also provides empirical evidence on the adaptability of RIAS in its application to an underexplored medical context, TCM encounters.

The survey findings indicate a greater patient-centeredness in TCM than in WM encounters. Most importantly, the results suggest a strong patient dissatisfaction with WM doctors in relation to their overwhelming talk about diagnostic testing, which could have important implications for health practitioners in WM practice. Doctors need to strike a balance between arranging for diagnostic testing and attending to patients' narration within a limited consultation time. Training programs on communication skills such as attentive listening might be helpful.

The three CA-informed studies provide empirical evidence on the interactional organizations in and through which these activities are accomplished. Examining the sequential environments of different activities helps us better understand the functions of these activities in the here-and-now interaction. Using CA, I have shown how the participants design their turns at talk in a sequence and how such a sequence instantiates an activity. These findings have implications for research and training. The results would be insightful for communication scholars and linguists who are interested in the language resources through which an activity is realized. For example, social scientists and health practitioners alike have considered that medical openings usually start with some form of phatic communion like the greeting sequence (Burnard, 2003; Coupland et al., 1992, 1994; Rinstedt, 2014). In contrast, Chapter 7 reported an absence of small talk in any form in WM conversations. This finding, therefore, poses challenges to the conventional belief that medical openings usually start with some formulaic expressions such as *how-are-you*. A similar finding to the present absence of phatic communion in the opening phase was reported in a Korean dental encounter (Park, 2021).

8.4.2 A longitudinal study of routine encounters

As highlighted at the beginning of the book and also in Chapter 2, most CA studies in this area have focused on acute care visits, primarily in the United Kingdom, the United States, and some European countries like Finland and Netherlands. Knowledge about what goes on in routine chronic encounters is scarce. Yet, chronic disease is the primary cause of mortality worldwide (WHO, 2003). Therefore, communication in such encounters is subject to comprehensive analysis.

In Chapter 1, I introduced the differences between TCM and WM in relation to their diagnostic approaches and their various pathologies in understanding disease. I mentioned the concept of 'medical formula' (Xue & O'Brien, 2003, p. 23), the prototypical TCM prescription recipe consisting of various herbs with separate but complementary functions. Normally, a recipe is designed for less than seven days. A patient needs to see the doctor several times to finish the whole course of treatment. In that sense, TCM consultations require a continuous progression of treatment. As Gu (1996) and Randel and Soong (1983) put it, a complete TCM treatment usually takes several continuous visits to finish the whole process. Future research could possibly recruit patients from their initial visit to the visit for which the current treatment counts as a complete one.

Chapter 5 explored how diagnostic testing is recommended in WM conversations, and I showed how it is used to disattend or postpone other interactional activities. Specifically, I presented examples when it makes relevant a temporary closing or interruption of the ongoing interaction. Due to practical concerns, I was unable to collect the follow-up interactions of those visits. A longitudinal study should allow us to understand how diagnostic test reports help doctors accomplish unfinished tasks, which can further substantiate, extend, and challenge the present findings.

8.4.3 *Communication in other modalities*

It is well known that video-recorded data provide more information than audio recordings, as much of the communication is nonverbal. This is particularly the case in medical consultations, where there is more than a factual presentation of problems. For example, Heath (1989, 2002) discussed how pain and suffering can be expressed by both verbal complaints and body conduct in medical consultations. The most recent developments in using video-based ethnographic and conversation analytic (EMCA) approaches to analyze various behaviors in healthcare settings have provided empirical evidence on the value of vocal and nonvocal conduct in understanding the practicalities of medical work (Heath et al., 2007; Parry, 2010). As Stivers and Sidnell (2005) suggested, the understanding of social interaction is based on the knowledge of how different modalities work together and the mechanisms underlying such cooperation. Studies use video-recorded data to analyze various activities such as problem elicitation (Robinson & Heritage, 2016), diagnosis (Heritage & McArthur, 2019; Peräkylä, 2010), the negotiating of informed choice (Zayts & Schnurr, 2011), and delivery of bad news (Kawashima, 2017).

I discussed in Chapter 4 how patients evaluate their doctors' performance across six domains of relational communication. A review of the literature suggests that a large number of relational messages (e.g., rapport and dominance) are delivered via nonverbal behaviors such as vocal sounds, gestures, and facial expressions (Robinson, 2006a). For example, Robinson (1998) discussed how doctors' and patients' gaze and body orientation reflect their level of engagement in medical consultations. Hillen et al. (2015) found that oncologists' eye contact is positively associated with patient trust, whereas smiling conveys friendliness and caring. Returning to the findings of Chapter 4, analysis based on video-recordings would be most useful for investigating doctors' performance in different domains of relational communication. Taking listening as an example, the findings in Chapter 4 suggest that doctors in WM encounters were less attentive to their patients than TCM doctors. With video-recordings, much can be gained from examining how the doctor disattends to the patient's turn-at-talk where it is situated visually and prosodically.

References

Atkinson, J. M., & Heritage, J. (Eds., 1984). *Structures of social action: Studies in conversation analysis.* Cambridge: Cambridge University Press.

Benwell, B., & McCreaddie, M. (2016). Keeping 'small talk' small in healthcare encounters: Negotiating the boundaries between on- and off-task talk. *Research on Language and Social Interaction, 49*(3), 258–271. https://doi.org/10.1080/08351813.2016.1196548

Burnard, P. (2003). Ordinary chat and therapeutic conversation: Phatic communication and mental health nursing. *Journal of Psychiatric and Mental Health Nursing, 10*(6), 678–682. https://doi.org/10.1046/j.1365-2850.2003.00639.x

Coupland, J., Coupland, N., & Robinson, J. D. (1992). 'How are you?': Negotiating phatic communion. *Language in Society, 21*(2), 207–230. https://doi.org/10.1017/S0047404500015268

Coupland, J., Robinson, J. D., & Coupland, N. (1994). Frame negotiation in doctor-elderly patient consultations. *Discourse & Society, 5*(1), 89–124. https://doi.org/10.1177%2F0957926594005001005

Cyranoski, D. (2018). Why Chinese medicine is heading for clinics around the world. *Nature, 561*, 448–450. https://doi.org/10.1038/d41586-018-06782-7

Deveugele, M., Derese, A., van den Brink-Muinen, A., Bensing, J., & de Maeseneer, J. (2002). Consultation length in general practice: Cross sectional study in six European countries. *BMJ, 325*(7362), 472. https://dx.doi.org/10.1136%2Fbmj.325.7362.472

Fu, Y., Schwebel, D. C., & Hu, G. (2018). Physicians' workloads in China: 1998–2016. *International Journal of Environmental Research and Public Health, 15*(8), 1649. https://doi.org/10.3390/ijerph15081649

Geraghty, E. M., Franks, P., & Kravitz, R. L. (2007). Primary care visit length, quality, and satisfaction for standardized patients with depression. *Journal of General Internal Medicine, 22*(12), 1641–1647. https://dx.doi.org/10.1007%2Fs11606-007-0371-5

Gu, Y. G. (1996). Doctor–patient interaction as goal-directed discourse in Chinese sociocultural context. *Journal of Asian Pacific Communication, 7*, 156–176.

Gude, T., Vaglum, P., Anvik, T., Bærheim, A., & Grimstad, H. (2013). A few more minutes make a difference? The relationship between content and length of GP consultations. *Scandinavian Journal of Primary Health Care, 31*(1), 31–35. https://doi.org/10.3109/02813432.2012.751698

Heath, C. (1989). Pain talk: The expression of suffering in the medical consultation. *Social Psychology Quarterly, 52*(2), 113–125. https://doi.org/10.2307/2786911

Heath, C. (2002). Demonstrative suffering: The gestural (re)embodiment of symptoms. *Journal of Communication, 52*(3), 597–616. https://doi.org/10.1111/j.1460-2466.2002.tb02564.x

Heath, C., Luff, P., & Svensson, M. S. (2007). Video and qualitative research: Analyzing medical practice and interaction. *Medical Education, 41*(1), 109–116. https://doi.org/10.1111/j.1365-2929.2006.02641.x

Heritage, J., & McArthur, A. (2019). The diagnostic moment: A study in US primary care. *Social Science & Medicine, 228*, 262–271. https://doi.org/10.1016/j.socscimed.2019.03.022

Hillen, M. A., de Haes, H. C. J. M., van Tienhoven, G., Bijker, N., van Laarhoven, H. W. M., Vermeulen, D. M., & Smets, E. M. A. (2015). All eyes on the patient: the influence of oncologists' nonverbal communication on breast cancer patients' trust. *Breast Cancer Research and Treatment, 153*, 161–171. https://doi.org/10.1007/s10549-015-3486-0

Howie, J. G., Hopton, J. L., Heaney, D. J., & Porter, A. M. D. (1992). Attitudes to medical care, the organisation of work, and stress among general practitioners. *British Journal of General Practice, 42*(358), 181–185.

Howie, J. G., Porter, A. M. D., Heaney, D. J., & Hopton, J. L. (1991). Long to short consultation ratio: A proxy measure of quality of care for general practice. *British Journal of General Practice, 41*(343), 48–54.

Hu, Y-H., & Zhang, Z-x. (2015). Skilled doctors in tertiary hospitals are already overworked in China. *The Lancet Global Health, 3*(12), e737. https://doi.org/10.1016/S2214-109X(15)00192-8

Irving, G., Neves, A. L., Dambha-Miller, H., Oishi, A., Tagashira, H., Verho, A., & Holden, J. (2017). International variations in primary care physician consultation time: a systematic review of 67 countries. *BMJ Open, 7*, e017902. https://doi.org/10.1136/bmjopen-2017-017902

Kawashima, M. (2017). Four ways of delivering very bad news in a Japanese emergency room. *Research on Language and Social Interaction, 50*(3), 307–325. https://doi.org/10.1080/08351813.2017.1340724

Maynard, D. W., & Hudak, P. L. (2008). Small talk, high stakes: Interactional disattentiveness in the context of prosocial doctor–patient interaction. *Language in Society, 37*(5), 661–688. https://doi.org/10.1017/S0047404508080986

Mishler, E. G. (1984). *The discourse of medicine: Dialectics of medical interviews.* Norwood, NJ: Ablex Publishing.

Orton, P. K. & Gray, D. P. (2016). Factors influencing consultation length in general/family practice. *Family Practice, 33*(5), 529–534. https://doi.org/10.1093/fampra/cmw056

Park, S. H. (2021). The dentist's first turn-at-talk in Korean dental visits. *Journal of Pragmatics, 185*, 1–14. https://doi.org/10.1016/j.pragma.2021.08.011

Parry, R. (2010). Video-based conversation analysis. In I. Bourgeault, R. Dingwall, & R. de Vries (Eds.), *The SAGE handbook of qualitative methods in health research* (pp. 373–396). Thousand Oaks, CA and London: Sage. https://dx.doi.org/10.4135/9781446268247.n20

Peräkylä, A. (2010). Agency and authority: Extended responses to diagnostic statements in primary care encounters. *Research on Language and Social Interaction, 35*(2), 219–247. https://doi.org/10.1207/S15327973RLSI3502_5

Prince, M. J., Wu, F., Guo, Y., Robledo, L. M. G., O'Donnell, M., Sullivan, R., & Yusuf, S. (2015). The burden of disease in older people and implications for health policy and practice. *The Lancet, 385*(9967), 549–562. https://doi.org/10.1016/S0140-6736(14)61347-7

Randel, S., & Soong, L. L. (1983). Traditional Chinese medicine in China. *The Western Journal of Medicine, 139*(2), 236–238.

Rinstedt, C. (2014). Conversational openings and multiparty disambiguations in doctors' encounters with young patients (and their parents). *Text & Talk, 34*(4), 421–442. https://doi.org/10.1515/text-2014-0010

Robinson, J. D. (1998). Getting down to business: Talk, gaze, and body orientation during openings of doctor–patient consultations. *Human Communication Research, 25*(1), 97–123. https://doi.org/10.1111/j.1468-2958.1998.tb00438.x

Robinson, J. D. (2006). Nonverbal communication and physician-patient inter-action: Review and new directions. In V. Manusov & M. L. Patterson (Eds.), *The SAGE handbook of nonverbal communication* (pp. 437–459). Thousand Oaks, CA and London: Sage. https://psycnet.apa.org/doi/10.4135/9781412976152.n23

Robinson, J. D., & Heritage, J. (2016). How patients understand physicians' solicitations of additional concerns: Implications for up-front agenda setting in primary care. *Health Communication, 31*(4), 434–444. https://doi.org/10.1080/10410236.2014.960060

Roter, D. L., Stewart, M., Putnam, S. M., Lipkin, M., Stiles, W. B., & Inui, T. S. (1997). Communication patterns of primary care physicians. *JAMA, 277*(4), 350–356.

Stivers, T., & Sidnell, J. (2005). Introduction: Multimodal interaction. *Semiotica, 156*(1/4), 1–20. https://doi.org/10.1515/semi.2005.2005.156.1

Tang, C., Liu, C., Fang, P., Xiang, Y., & Min, R. (2019). Work-related accumulated fatigue among doctors in tertiary hospitals: A cross-sectional survey in six provinces of China. *International Journal of Environmental Research and Public Health, 16*(17), 3049. https://doi.org/10.3390/ijerph16173049

Taylor, K. (2009). Paternalism, participation and partnership – The evolution of patient centeredness in the consultation. *Patient Education and Counseling, 74*(2), 150–155. https://doi.org/10.1016/j.pec.2008.08.017

Tu, J., Wang, C., & Wu, S. (2015). Skilled doctors in tertiary hospitals are already overworked in China – Author's reply. *The Lancet Global Health, 3*(12), E738. https://doi.org/10.1016/S2214-109X(15)00190-4

Wilson, A., & Childs, S. (2002). The relationship between consultation length, process and outcomes in general practice: A systematic review. *British Journal of General Practice, 52*(485), 1012–1020.

World Health Organization (2003). *Diet, nutrition, and the prevention of chronic diseases: Report of a joint WHO/FAO expert consultation.* Technical Report Series No. 916. Geneva: WHO. https://apps.who.int/nutrition/publications/obesity/WHO_TRS_916/en/

Xue, C. C., & O'Brien, K. A. (2003). Modalities of Chinese medicine. In P. C. Leung, C. C. Xue, & Y. C. Cheng (Eds.), *A comprehensive guide to Chinese medicine* (pp. 19–46). Hackensack, NJ: World Scientific. https://doi.org/10.1142/9789812794987_0002

Zayts, O., & Schnurr, S. (2011). Laughter as medical providers' resource: Negotiating informed choice in prenatal genetic counseling. *Research on Language and Social Interaction, 44*(1), 1–20. https://doi.org/10.1080/08351813.2011.544221

Index

For Product Safety Concerns and Information please contact our EU
representative GPSR@taylorandfrancis.com
Taylor & Francis Verlag GmbH, Kaufingerstraße 24, 80331 München, Germany